Contents

A Guide to Laboratory

Radcliffe Publishing
London • New York

Radcliffe Publishing Ltd
St Mark's House
Shepherdess Walk
London N1 7LH
United Kingdom

www.radcliffehealth.com

First edition 1989
Second edition 1993
Third edition 2000
Fourth edition 2003
Fifth edition 2008

Michael McGhee has asserted his right under the Copyright, Designs and Patents Act 1988 to be identified as the author of this work.

New research and clinical experience can result in changes in treatment and drug therapy. Readers of this book should therefore check the most recent product information on any drug they may prescribe to ensure they are complying with the manufacturer's recommendations concerning dosage, the method and duration of administration, and contraindications. Every effort has been made to ensure that the information in this book is accurate. This does not diminish the requirement to exercise clinical judgement, and neither the publisher nor the author can accept any responsibility for its use in practice.

British Library Cataloguing in Publication Data

A catalogue record for this book is available from the British Library.

ISBN-13: 978 190891 153 7

The paper used for the text pages of this book is FSC® certified. FSC (The Forest Stewardship Council®) is an international network to promote responsible management of the world's forests.

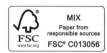

Typeset by Darkriver Design, Auckland, New Zealand
Printed and bound by TJ International Ltd, Padstow, Cornwall, UK

Preface

In the 6 years since the last edition of this book was published, much more patient care has become the responsibility of doctors in primary care. Laboratory testing, to establish a diagnosis, monitor response to treatment and manage the ongoing care of the patient is now within the domain of primary care more than ever before. In the UK approximately 700 million laboratory tests are processed annually at a cost of more than £2.5 billion. Since the establishment of clinical commissioning groups, the cost of laboratory investigations is under closer scrutiny than ever before. A basic full blood count costs around £10, liver function tests around £10, urea and electrolytes around £7 and thyroid function tests around £20. Making appropriate decisions on when and how to interpret tests is therefore more important than ever. Some older established tests, such as prostate-specific antigen, CA 125 and other tumour markers and HbA$_{1c}$, are being used and interpreted differently and newer more specific tests such as anti-citrullinated peptide is now more readily available in primary care to detect rheumatoid arthritis. Authorities such as the National Institute for Health and Care Excellence regularly advise doctors to monitor patients – particularly those with chronic diseases – more than ever before. Since the last edition of this book new sections have been added, including suggestions for appropriate laboratory tests in certain clinical situations, e.g. dementia screen, screening tests when a patient presents with a neuropathy, and appropriate tests for patients presenting with hypertension, chronic fatigue syndrome, erectile dysfunction, gynaecomastia and several other common presentations in primary care.

This concise text attempts to address all of the questions arising from the interpretation of normal and abnormal laboratory tests. It is written by a full-time practising GP and trainer who is constantly alert to laboratory tests, both new and old, and how to make the most of them and interpret them properly in general practice. The information should be of use to the doctor and his or her practice nurse, both in primary care and in out-of-hours care settings.

Michael McGhee
September 2013

Glossary

ACE	angiotensin-converting enzyme
ACR	albumin/creatinine ratio
AF	atrial fibrillation
AFP	alpha-fetoprotein
AIDS	acquired immune deficiency syndrome
ALOs	*Actinomyces*-like organisms
ALP	alkaline phosphatase
ALT	alanine transferase
Amp-C	Amp C beta-lactamase producers
ANA	antinuclear antibody
ANCA	antineutrophil cytoplasmic antibody
APC-R	activated protein C resistance
AS	antistreptolysin-O
AST	aspartate transferase
BNP	B-type natriuretic peptide
BP	blood pressure
CHD	coronary heart disease
CIN	cervical intra-epithelial neoplasia
CK	creatine kinase
CKD	chronic kidney disease
CLL	chronic lymphatic leukaemia
CREST	calcinosis, Raynaud's phenomenon, oesophageal dysmotility, sclerodactyly, telangiectasia
CRP	C-reactive protein
CSF	cerebrospinal fluid
CTD	connective tissue disease
DAT	differential agglutination test
DEXA	dual energy X-ray absorptiometry
DIC	disseminated intravascular coagulation
DMARD	disease-modifying anti-rheumatic drug
DNA	deoxyribonucleic acid
dsDNA	double-stranded DNA
DVT	deep vein thrombosis
EBV	Epstein–Barr virus

ECG	electrocardiograph
EDTA	ethylenediaminetetra-acetic acid
eGFR	estimated glomerular filtration rate
ESBL	extended-spectrum beta-lactamase
ESR	erythrocyte sedimentation rate
FAI	free androgen index
FBC	full blood count
FH	familial hyperlipidaemia
FOB	faecal occult blood
FSH	follicle-stimulating hormone
FTAABS	fluorescent treponemal antibody absorption test
GBM	glomerular basement membrane
GGT	gamma-glutamyl transferase
GPL	G phospholipid
Hb	haemoglobin
HCG	human chorionic gonadotrophin
HDL	high-density lipoprotein
HDN	haemolytic disease of the newborn
HIV	human immunodeficiency virus
HLA	human leucocyte antigen
HPV	human papilloma virus
HVA	homovanillic acid
HVS	high vaginal swab
IgA	immunoglobulin A
IgE	immunoglobulin E
IGF-1	insulin-like growth factor-1
IgG	immunoglobulin G
IgM	immunoglobulin M
INR	international normalised ratio
IUCD	intrauterine contraceptive device
KCCT	kaolin cephalin clotting time
LAD	left axis deviation
LBBB	left bundle branch block
LDH	lactic dehydrogenase
LDL	low-density lipoprotein
LFT	liver function test
LH	luteinising hormone
LVH	left ventricular hypertrophy
MCH	mean corpuscular haemoglobin
MCHC	mean corpuscular haemoglobin concentration
MCV	mean corpuscular volume
MDS	myelodysplastic syndrome

MGUS	monoclonal gammopathy of undetermined significance
MI	myocardial infarction
MSU	mid-stream urine specimen
nocte	at night
NSAID	non-steroidal anti-inflammatory drug
od	once daily
PA	pernicious anaemia
PCOS	polycystic ovarian syndrome
PCR	protein/creatinine ratio
PCV	packed cell volume
PE	pulmonary embolism
PMR	polymyalgia rheumatic
PPI	proton pump inhibitor
PRV	polycythaemia rubra vera
PSA	prostate-specific antigen
qid	*quater in die* – four times a day
RA	rheumatoid arthritis
RAHA	rheumatoid arthritis haemagglutination assay
RBC	red blood cell count
SCAT	sheep cell agglutination test
SHBG	sex-hormone-binding globulin
SIADH	syndrome of inappropriate antidiuretic hormone
SLE	systemic lupus erythematosus
T$_3$	tri-iodothyronine
T$_4$	thyroxine
TB	tuberculosis
TBG	thyroxine-binding globulin
TC	total cholesterol
tds	*ter in die* – three times a day
TFT	thyroid function test
TG	triglyceride
TIBC	total iron-binding capacity
TPO	thyroid peroxidase
TSH	thyroid-stimulating hormone
U&E	urea and electrolytes test
UTI	urinary tract infection
VDRL	Venereal Disease Reference Laboratory
VMA	vanillylmandelic acid
WBC	white blood cell count
WCC	white cell count

Ca^{2+}	calcium
Cl^-	chloride
Cu^{2+}	copper
dl	decilitre
fl	femtolitre
g	gram
IU	international unit
IV	intravenous
K^+	potassium
kU	kilo-unit
l	litre
Li^+	lithium
mEq	milli-equivalent
mg	milligram
Mg^{2+}	magnesium
µg	microgram
µmol	micromole
mIU	milli-international unit
ml	millilitre
mm	millimetre
mmHg	millimetres of mercury pressure
mmol	millimole
mU	milli-unit
Na^+	sodium
ng	nanogram
nmol	nanomole
pg	picogram
pmol	picomole
U	unit
Zn^{2+}	zinc
%	percentage
<	less than
=	equals
>	more than
≥	more than or equal to

Introduction

CONSULTATION AND REFERRAL

General practitioners vary in their use of the laboratory services, with variation of up to tenfold between comparable practices in the rates of blood tests requested per patient. Variation occurs not only in the use of the pathology and radiology facilities, but also in the use of specialist referral.

Although many investigations are performed in order to confirm or refute a clinical suspicion (e.g. anaemia or hypothyroidism), an increasing number of tests are conducted as part of screening (e.g. Well Man and Well Woman screening clinics). Because investigations are used in this way, and as reports contain more information than is requested, unexpected findings (e.g. mild thrombocytopenia) are not uncommon.

The GP then has to decide whether to react to the test or ignore it, if it is not significantly outside the normal range. While many laboratories publish a guide to their own local laboratory values, which may vary according to the technique employed by the laboratory, it is left to the clinician who is requesting the test to decide on appropriate action as a result of the test.

The intention of this desktop-ready reference is to help practitioners to make a more informed choice with regard to further investigation or referral as appropriate, and to prompt further investigations if they would be helpful. There will never be any substitute for a good clinical history and thorough physical examination, but this book will, it is hoped, fill in some of the blanks when an appropriate history, examination and investigations have taken place.

Chapter 1

Haematology

CASES THAT THE HAEMATOLOGIST MUST SEE

There are a number of haematological conditions that must be referred to a consultant.

The following unexpected haematological findings *should be referred immediately*.

- Abnormal blood films, such as abnormal, immature or odd-shaped cells, are always commented on by the haematologist, who will usually indicate that referral is necessary.

- Haemoglobin (Hb) >19 (male) or >17 (female) g/dl or <8.5 g/dl.

- White blood cell count (WCC) <2.0 or >25 × 10^9/l.

- Neutrophil count <0.5 × 10^9/l.

- Platelets <80 × 10^9/l.

- Refractory anaemia (i.e. anaemia that fails to respond to haematinics).

- Obscure anaemias (e.g. those where the blood film carries a comment such as 'spherocytes seen').

- Haemoglobinopathies and thalassaemias. Remember that an unexplained hypochromic microcytic anaemia may well represent thalassaemia and not iron deficiency.

- Suspected bleeding disorders such as clotting defects.

RED CELL INDICES
Hb

A recent national harmonisation programme initiated by the Department of Health has resulted in Hb and mean corpuscular haemoglobin concentration (MCHC) being reported in grams per litre instead of grams per decilitre, so a Hb of 13.5 g/dl becomes 135 g/l.

In an individual, the Hb level remains fairly constant, but between individuals there may be variation of up to 30 g/l.

- A reduction in plasma volume caused by dehydration or strenuous muscular exercise may increase the Hb by up to 15 g/l.

- A 5–10% drop in Hb may be seen on assuming a lying position from standing.

- Normal range (g/l) for adults:

  - male, 133–180

  - female, 115–165.

- Normal range (g/l) for children:

  - at birth, 165 (135–195)

  - 2 weeks, 165 (125–205)

  - 2 months, 115 (90–140)

  - 6 months, 115 (95–135)

  - puberty (male), 130–160

  - puberty (female), 120–160.

Abnormal test results
- Raised Hb suggests:

  - polycythaemia (raised Hb, raised haematocrit or packed cell volume (PCV) and total red blood cell count (RBC) raised)

  - smoking (increases the Hb due to increased carboxyhaemoglobin)

  - hypoxia and some renal conditions in which excess erythropoietin is produced.

Smoking increases the Hb level in direct proportion to the number of cigarettes smoked.

- Lowered Hb indicates anaemia. In young females the most common cause is heavy menstrual loss. Other red cell indices can help to identify the likely cause of anaemia. Clinical symptoms of anaemia often do not appear until the Hb level has fallen to 70–90 g/l.

RBC

- Male, $4.0–5.9 \times 10^{12}/l$
- Female, $3.8–5.2 \times 10^{12}/l$
- High RBCs seen in polycythaemia and in dehydration.
- Low RBCs seen in any cause of anaemia and thalassaemia.

Haematocrit or PCV (MCV multiplied by RBC)

- Normal range (ml) for adults:
  - male, 0.40–0.54 (41–54%)
  - female, 0.35–0.47 (35–47%).
- Normal range (ml) for children:
  - at birth, 0.42–0.54
  - 1–3 years, 0.29–0.4
  - 4–10 years, 0.36–0.38.
- Raised levels indicate: increased red blood cell production (e.g. chronic hypoxia associated with pulmonary disease and congenital heart disease), polycythaemia rubra vera (PRV) or lowered plasma volume (e.g. dehydration, stress polycythaemia or pseudopolycythaemia).
- Lowered PCV is found in acute blood volume loss, anaemia and overhydration.
- PCV of >0.45 is strongly associated with thromboembolic disease.
- PCV of >0.52 should always be investigated.

Polycythaemia

- PCV of >0.48 in females.
- PCV of >0.51 in males.

- Hypertension, smoking and stress can cause stress polycythaemia or pseudopolycythaemia.

- In primary polycythaemia (previously know as PRV) Hb is raised, haematocrit or PCV is raised and RBC is raised.

- In PRV, as well as the red cell changes, the white cell count (WCC) and platelet count are also raised.

- Pseudopolycythaemia or stress polycythaemia is characterised by a raised Hb level, a normal WCC, normal platelet count, normal red cell mass and decreased plasma volume.

- In the treatment of polycythaemia by venesection, the aim is to achieve a target haematocrit (PCV) of 0.45.

- Up to 15% of patients with PRV will eventually develop a form of leukaemia that is often resistant to chemotherapy.

Mean corpuscular volume (MCV)

- Normal range (fl) is 80–99, although it is lower in children (78 at age 1 year). The mean cell volume increases with age in males.

Abnormal test results

- Raised MCV suggests:
  - vitamin B_{12} or folate deficiency (either dietary or due to malabsorption)
  - myxoedema, alcohol or liver disease
  - occasionally aplastic anaemia and myelodysplasias haemolysis aplasia or marrow infiltration.

- Vitamin B_{12} and/or folate deficiency both cause a raised MCV, usually accompanied by a low Hb, low white cell count and low platelets.

- After 3 months (the lifespan of the red blood cell) the MCV should return to normal. Its failure to do so warrants further investigation, e.g. thyroid function tests or bone marrow examination for myelodysplasia.

- Checking the reticulocyte count after commencing B_{12} or folate replacement confirms new red blood cell production in response to treatment.

- Lowered MCV (microcytosis) suggests:

    - chronic blood loss, commonly menstrual in young females or occult blood loss due to gastrointestinal disease in older patients

    - iron-deficiency anaemia

    - thalassaemia

    - sideroblastic anaemia (myelodysplastic syndrome)

    - anaemia of chronic disease.

- Microcytosis, especially in the absence of anaemia, is strongly suggestive of the thalassaemia trait, especially in patients of foreign origin. Electrophoresis will usually show a raised HbA_2 unless there is a coexisting iron deficiency.

- The MCV may be normal in anaemia of chronic disease, uraemia, acute blood loss, myeloproliferative disorders and bone marrow infiltration, or where vitamin B_{12} or folate deficiency are combined with iron deficiency or thalassaemia.

Mean corpuscular haemoglobin (MCH)

- Normal range (pg) is 27–33.

- The MCH and MCHC should not be interpreted alone but in conjunction with the other red cell parameters.

Abnormal test results

- Raised MCH suggests:

    - vitamin B_{12} or folate deficiency, myxoedema.

- Lowered MCH suggests:

    - iron deficiency

    - thalassaemia

    - chronic blood loss

    - megaloblastic anaemia.

MCHC

- Normal range (g/l) is 320–360.

Abnormal test results

- Lowered MCHC suggests:
  - iron deficiency
  - blood loss.
- Raised MCHC may be seen in the presence of spherocytes and sickle cells.

Activated protein C resistance (APC-R)

- Activated protein C resistance is an inherited condition characterised by factor V being abnormally resistant to degradation by activated protein C, resulting in a tendency for blood to clot more easily.

- The gene responsible for APC-R was discovered in 1994 in Leiden, the Netherlands, and is often called factor V Leiden.

- APC-R is probably the commonest inherited condition known, affecting 5–8% of the population.

- Anyone with APC-R has a 50% chance of a brother or sister having it, and will have one parent who has it.

- Some patients may have a double dose of APC-R, if both parents have the gene, and are therefore at even greater risk of blood clots.

- The normal range of APC-R is 2.2–7.0.

Abnormal test results

A low test result indicates a higher-than-normal likelihood of thrombosis. High-oestrogen oral contraceptive pills should be avoided. Prophylaxis against thrombosis should be considered in major surgery.

Anti-cardiolipin IgG

Anti-cardiolipin IgG is an antibody against the beta-2 glycoprotein coagulation system. A significantly raised level is indicative of an increased risk of thrombosis, and is often found in autoimmune disease and in patients with recurrent miscarriages (more than three), and is thought to be due to placental thrombosis.

- The results for levels of cardiolipin antibodies should be interpreted with caution.

- Low positive levels may be found in normal people.

- Interpretive guidelines:

  - normal, ≤7.2 U/ml

  - negative, <13.3

  - low positive, 13.4–19.9

  - moderate, 20–80

  - high, >80.1.

ANAEMIA
Common causes of anaemia
Anaemia with decreased MCV
This may be due to:
  - iron deficiency

  - thalassaemia and some haemoglobinopathies

  - anaemia of chronic disease.

- Further investigations:

  - blood film

  - serum ferritin (the most useful test for iron deficiency)

  - electrophoresis

  - reticulocyte count

  - faecal occult blood.

Anaemia with normal MCV
This may be due to:
  - acute blood loss

  - haemolysis

  - anaemia of chronic disease

  - chronic renal disease

- haemoglobinopathy
- bone marrow failure (e.g. aplastic anaemia or leukaemia).

- Further investigations:
  - blood film
  - reticulocyte count
  - electrophoresis
  - serum ferritin (the most useful test for iron deficiency)
  - serum vitamin B_{12}
  - serum and red cell folate
  - renal function tests
  - serum bilirubin.

Anaemia with an elevated MCV

This may be due to:
- megaloblastic anaemia, vitamin B_{12} deficiency or folate deficiency
- non-megaloblastic causes (e.g. liver disease, thyroid disease, alcohol, reticulocytosis, myelodysplasia).

- Further investigations:
  - blood film
  - serum vitamin B_{12}
  - serum and red cell folate
  - liver function tests
  - thyroid function tests.

- Iron deficiency is the commonest cause of anaemia in the UK.

- Chronic illness may be the most common cause of anaemia in the elderly.

- Slow-release iron preparations should not be used to treat anaemia.

- Failure of anaemia to respond to treatment may be due to lack of compliance.

Haemolytic anaemia

- Haemolysis in the presence of anaemia can be confirmed by the presence of large numbers of reticulocytes on the blood film, and a raised serum bilirubin level.

Serum ferritin

- This is an iron–protein complex that plays a part in absorption, transport and storage.

- Serum iron and total iron-binding capacity (TIBC) have been largely superceded by serum ferritin.

- Normal range (µg/l):

  - adult male, 30–300

  - pre-menopausal female, 7–280

  - post-menopausal female, 14–230

  - children aged 6 months to 15 years, 7–150.

- Serum ferritin is influenced by diet and recent oral therapy.

Abnormal test results

- Low serum ferritin indicates iron deficiency.

- Lowered serum ferritin, and lowered folate and low vitamin B_{12} suggest malabsorption.

- Normal or raised serum ferritin suggests:

  - liver disease

  - malignancy

  - chronic inflammation (e.g. rheumatoid arthritis (RA)) (yet the iron and TIBC may be reduced).

- Raised serum ferritin may be indicative of haemochromatosis, an inborn error of iron metabolism, which may present with vague symptoms, e.g. weakness, lethargy, loss of libido, impotence or weight loss. Organ damage is likely if undetected, e.g. liver damage (cirrhosis/hepatocellular cancer), pancreas (diabetes), arthropathy (chondrocalcinosis), abnormal skin pigmentation, cardiomyopathy and gonadal hypertrophy can all occur.

NB: The lower limit of the normal ferritin range is raised in chronic disease (e.g. RA with ferritin of 40 is probably iron deficient).

Serum iron

- Normal range (µg%) is 80–150.

- Ideally, blood should be taken in a fasting state and not while the patient is taking oral iron.

- This is a cheaper investigation than serum ferritin, but gives a less accurate indication of body iron stores.

Abnormal test results

- Lowered serum iron and lowered TIBC with normal or raised ferritin suggest anaemia of chronic disease.

- Increased serum iron is seen in:
  - iron overload
  - contraceptive pill users
  - liver disease anaemias (e.g. haemolysis)
  - haemochromatosis (raised iron, raised serum ferritin, reduced TIBC).

- Haemochromatosis is part of the differential diagnosis in the investigation of abnormal LFT. All first-degree relatives of patients with haemochromatosis should be screened for the disease by genetic testing for the HFE genotype.

- Hb and iron levels in pregnancy:
  - Hb <11.0 g/dl at first contact or <10.5 at 28 weeks should be investigated and iron supplementation given if appropriate. In late pregnancy, Hb <10 g/dl should be referred to an obstetrician for further management.

- Iron-binding capacity (25–60 µmol/l) is reduced in:
  - iron-deficiency anaemia
  - chronic infection
  - malignancy
  - hypothyroidism

- and raised in:
  - haemolytic, megaloblastic and aplastic anaemia
  - thalassaemia
  - lead poisoning.

Iron-deficiency anaemia

- This is characterised by low ferritin, low serum iron, raised TIBC, low MCV and low MCHC.
- Blood film may show hypochromasia, anisocytosis, poikilocytosis and pencil cells.
- MCV falls in parallel with Hb and is often lower than in thalassaemia. RBC may be normal.
- Iron-deficiency anaemia may be caused by:
  - blood loss from the gastrointestinal tract
  - menorrhagia
  - pregnancy
  - malabsorption or dietary insufficiency.
- In the treatment of anaemia, the Hb should rise by 2 g/dl every 3 weeks. Its failure to do so should lead to the consideration of blood loss, malabsorption or poor compliance with treatment.
- Treatment of anaemia should continue for 3 months after the correction of the anaemia in order to replenish iron stores.
- Iron in the stool:
  - it is impossible in a patient who is taking oral iron to distinguish between the black stool due to the presence of iron and the black stool due to blood in the stool melaena, although the melaena stool is characteristically tarry and has a distinctive odour.

Normochromic normocytic anaemia

- This is characterised by low Hb, normal MCV, normal MCH and normal MCHC.
- It may be caused by:
  - chronic disorders (e.g. renal failure, RA)

- pregnancy
- recent blood loss
- haemolysis.
- Anaemia of chronic kidney disease (CKD)
  - Treatment of anaemia of CKD (which is more common in CKD stages 4 and 5 but can occur in stages 2 and 3) should be initiated in patients when the Hb is <11 g/dl (or <10 g/dl if age under 2 years) and should aim for a target Hb of between 10.5 and 12.5 g/dl for adults and children over age 2 years, and between 10 and 12 g/dl in children under age 2 years.

Haemolysis

- Haemolysis may be congenital, e.g.:
  - sickle-cell disease
  - thalassaemia
  - congenital spherocytosis
  - glucose-6-phosphate dehydrogenase deficiency causing haemolysis with certain drugs (e.g. sulphonamides, nitrofurantoin and quinine).
- Alternatively, it may be acquired, e.g.:
  - infections (e.g. mononucleosis, mycoplasma)
  - systemic lupus erythematosus (SLE)
  - drugs (e.g. penicillins, cephalosporin, quinine, methyldopa, hydralazine, antimalarials or sulphonamide antibiotics)
  - malignancy
  - endocrine deficiency
  - aplasia
  - systemic disease (e.g. liver disease, uraemia).

Macrocytic anaemia

- This is characterised by lowered Hb and MCV >99.
- As well as macrocytes in the blood film, additional features include

hypersegmentation of the neutrophils and occasionally leucopenia and thrombocytopenia.

- Macrocytic anaemia is often due to vitamin B_{12} or folate deficiency causing megaloblastic changes in the bone marrow. Vitamin B_{12} deficiency may be dietary in origin (e.g. in Hindu vegetarians, vegans) or due to pernicious anaemia. Folate deficiency may be due to malabsorption or antifolate drugs (e.g. anticonvulsants, trimethoprim or triamterene).

- Macrocytic anaemia may also be due to non-megaloblastic causes:

  - alcohol

  - liver disease

  - myxoedema

  - aplastic anaemia

  - myeloma.

Serum folate

- This is usually measured in conjunction with red cell folate.

- Normal range (µg/l) is 2–14 (5–40 nmol/l).

- Red cell folate is a better guide to tissue stores, while serum folate indicates the immediate level.

Red cell folate

- This is usually measured in conjunction with serum folate.

- Normal range (µg/l) is 130–620 (400–1600 nmol/l).

- Red cell folate may be low in vitamin B_{12} deficiency states, e.g. dietary malabsorption and antifolate drugs.

Vitamin B_{12}

- Normal range (ng/l) is 170–700.

- Low WCC can cause a low B_{12}.

- In pernicious anaemia (PA), levels are often <50.

- 10–15% of people with PA have normal vitamin B_{12} levels.

- Normal range (IU/ml) is <2.5.

Serum intrinsic factor antibody assay
Abnormal test results
- Lowered serum intrinsic factor antibody assay (<2) suggests a negative result.

- A borderline result (2.5) suggests that a repeat test should be performed.

- Raised serum intrinsic factor antibody assay (>2.5) suggests pernicious anaemia.

Reticulocyte count
- If anaemia is present, the reticulocyte count gives an indication of the marrow response.

- Normal range (%) is 0.2–2.

- Peaks occur 3–5 days after the start of treatment with folic acid or vitamin B_{12} and 7 days after treatment with iron.

Abnormal test results
- A raised reticulocyte count suggests:

  - haemolysis following haemorrhage

  - a response to treatment with haematinics.

Plasma viscosity
- Measures the flow rate of plasma compared with water.

- Normal range (mPa) is 1.25–1.72.

- Advantages of the plasma viscosity test over erythrocyte sedimentation rate (ESR):

  - it is independent of age, sex and Hb level

  - plasma can be kept at room temperature for 48 hours without affecting the result (unlike ESR, which must be read within 4 hours)

  - steroids *do not* affect the result

  - high sensitivity, few false-negative results

  - the test is easily automated

  - it is cheap.

Test results

- Reduced plasma viscosity (<1.5) occurs in low plasma proteins.

- Normal range is 1.5–1.72 (up to 1.8 in the third trimester of pregnancy).

- Raised plasma viscosity (1.72–3.0) occurs in acute or chronic disease.

- Raised plasma viscosity (>3.0) strongly suggests myeloma or macroglobulinaemia (levels usually greatly exceed this value).

Erythrocyte sedimentation rate (ESR)

- This measurement varies widely in different physiological and pathological conditions.

- The ESR is influenced by age, sex and anaemia and must be measured within 4 hours of venepuncture.

- The 'normal' range varies depending on the technique (e.g. Westergren, Wintrobe or Seditainer).

- The approximate normal range (using the Westergren method) for males is equal to the age in years divided by 2; and for females is equal to the age in years +10 divided by 2.

- The specimen should remain in a vertical position and must be transported to the laboratory immediately.

- If the specimen is refrigerated, it should be allowed to warm to room temperature before being tested.

Abnormal test results

- Raised ESR can be found in:
  - disease (any acute inflammatory response), e.g. temporal arteritis, though note that the ESR can be normal in temporal arteritis
  - pregnancy
  - oral contraceptive pill users
  - anaemia (falsely evelated result)
  - obsesity can cause a moderately raised ESR.

NB: Very high (>100) ESR is found in autoimmune disease; malignancy; acute post-trauma, and serious infection. A false high ESR can occur if the ambient temperature is unusually high; if the Westergren tube is not held vertically, or if dextran is present in the blood sample.

- Low ESR is found in:

  - heart failure

  - PRV

  - sickle-cell anaemia

  - treatment with steroids.

  NB: A false low ESR can occur if the ambient temperature is unusually low, if the Westergren tube contains air bubbles, or if the tube is dirty.

C-reactive protein (CRP)

- C-reactive protein is an acute phase protein, so it is elevated in infection (more so with bacterial infection, less elevated with viral infection) and inflammation but not elevated with many malignancies.

- Normal range (mg/l) is <4.

- It changes more rapidly than ESR.

- Levels are increased up to several hundred times following an acute infective or non-infective inflammatory response.

- Elevation may occur in lipaemic sera.

- CRP is sometimes used to monitor the response to second-line drugs in the treatment of RA. Maintaining CRP within the normal range leads to less joint erosion.

- CRP levels are often normal in malignancy.

Serum haptoglobin

- This is a serum protein which combines with Hb.

- Normal range (g/l) is 0.3–2.0.

- It is measured principally in patients in whom acute haemolysis is suspected, when levels may fall below 0.1.

- An increase in haptoglobin occurs in many systemic diseases and inflammatory conditions.

Infectious mononucleosis

- Infection with the Epstein–Barr virus (human herpes type 4 virus) has been implicated in a wide spectrum of clinical diseases, ranging from glandular fever to lymphoma.

- Diagnosis of glandular fever is by the following.

  - The *Monospot test* – a rapid, simple slide test for the detection of heterophil antibodies. It is less specific and less sensitive than the Paul–Bunnell test, giving negative results for 10–20% of adults with proven infectious mononucleosis and up to 50% of children.

- Atypical lymphocytes >10% are commonly but not always seen in glandular fever.

- Other viral infections that may cause a lymphocytosis, but which give a negative Paul–Bunnell test, include:

  - viral hepatitis

  - rubella

  - toxoplasmosis

  - cytomegalovirus infection

  - HIV infection.

- Liver function tests will often be abnormal in patients with glandular fever; transaminases and bilirubin levels reach 2–3 times normal in over 80% of patients with glandular fever.

WHITE CELL INDICES
WBC

- Normal range ($\times 10^9$/l) is 4–11.

- The WCC is similar in males and females, and remains very constant throughout life in 50% of the population.

- More important than the total WCC is the *differential white cell count*. WCCs of >11 $\times$ 10^9/l should have a differential WCC performed.

- The WCC rarely exceeds 50 $\times$ 10^9/l except in leukaemia.

- The total WBC or any individual element may be lowered by steroids.

  NB: Individuals of Afro-Caribbean origin have a lower normal range.

Differential WBC

- Normal range ($\times 10^9$/l):

    - neutrophils, 2.5–7.5 (60–70%)

    - lymphocytes, 1.5–4.0 (25–30%)

    - monocytes, 0.2–0.8 (5–10%)

    - eosinophils, 0.04–0.44 (1–4%)

    - basophils, up to 0.1 (up to 1%).

- Individuals of Afro-Caribbean origin have lower neutrophil counts than do individuals of other races.

- Neutrophil normal range, 2.5–7.5 $\times$ 10^9/l.

- Mild neutropenia, 1.0–2.5 $\times$ 10^9/l.

- Moderate neutropenia, 0.5–1.0 $\times$ 10^9/l.

- Severe neutropenia, <0.5 $\times$ 10^9/l.

- Neutrophil count <0.5: REFER IMMEDIATELY.

- Neutrophil count 0.5–1.0, repeat in 1 week if patient is well; if patient is unwell or febrile, ADMIT TO HOSPITAL.

- Neutrophil count 1.0–2.0, repeat in 4 weeks.

NB: Young children normally have a reverse differential count, i.e. more lymphocytes than neutrophils.

Abnormal test results

- Neutropenia (neutrophils $<1 \times 10^9/l$) may be due to:

  - infections (e.g. bacterial/viral tuberculosis (TB), typhoid, brucellosis, rickettsia and malaria)

  - autoimmune disorders, e.g. RA, SLE

  - haematological disorders, e.g. leukaemia, myelodysplasia, myeloma, lymphoma, vitamin B_{12} or folate deficiency

  - drugs (e.g. antibacterial drugs (e.g. penicillin, cephalosprins, doxycycline, trimethoprim, metronidazole), analgesics (e.g. aspirin, indomethacin, ibuprofen), psychiatric drugs (e.g. chlorpromazine, risperidone, chlordiazepoxide, mianserin), anticonvulsants (e.g. phenytoin, sodium valproate, carbamazepine), cytotoxic therapy, some antirheumatic agents (especially gold), cardiovascular drugs (e.g. propranolol, nifedipine, captopril, spironolactone), thiazide diuretics and many others, including colchicine, allopurinol, metoclopramide and carbimazole).

  - When referring routinely for a non-urgent haematolgy opinion (neutrophils <1 in a well patient), request antinuclear antibodies (ANA), LDH, B_{12} and folate and protein electrophoresis.

- Cigarette smokers often have high (but normal) white cell counts proportional to the number of cigarettes smoked, presumed to be due to inflammatory lung disease.

- Raised WBC (leucocytosis) is commonly found in:

  - bacterial infection

  - pregnancy (third trimester)

  - post-trauma (e.g. burns, surgery)

  - post-haemorrhage

  - malignancy

  - drugs (e.g. steroids, digoxin, lithium, beta-agonists)

  - myeloproliferative disorders

- myocardial infarction (MI)
- renal failure
- gout
- diabetes mellitus.
- A lowered white cell count necessitates a differential white cell count.
- The white cell count may be lowered in:
  - viral infections
  - bacterial infection (e.g. overwhelming septicaemia, brucellosis, typhoid, miliary tuberculosis)
  - drugs (e.g. thiouracil, mianserin, meprobamate and phenylbutazone)
  - folate or vitamin B_{12} deficiency
  - autoimmune neutropenia
  - SLE
  - Felty's syndrome
  - post-coronary artery bypass-graft
  - haemodialysis agranulocytosis (severe leucopenia in an ill patient).
- Agranulocytosis can be caused by:
  - drugs that give rise to pancytopenia (e.g. antimitotic drugs and antirheumatic drugs such as gold, as well as carbimazole)
  - some malignancies (e.g. leukaemia, non-Hodgkin's lymphoma) may present with low WBC.
- Eosinophils >6% (eosinophilia) suggests:
  - allergic reactions (e.g. to drugs, parasites)
  - polyarteritis
  - reticulocytosis
  - sarcoidosis
  - myeloproliferative disorders

- leukaemia
- erythema multiforme
- irradiation
- congenital causes
- dermatitis herpetiformis
- pemphigus
- scarlet fever
- acute rheumatic fever
- rheumatoid arthritis
- smoking.
- A very high eosinophil count is seen in some carcinomas, hydatid disease and eosinophilic leukaemia.
- A lowered eosinophil count occurs with corticosteroids and occurs during the early phase of acute insults and shock and trauma surgery.
- Lymphocytosis is defined as a lymphocyte count $>5 \times 10^9$/l.
- A lymphocyte count of >45% (lymphocytosis) is found in some infections (e.g. infectious mononucleosis, infectious hepatitis, cytomegalovirus, toxoplasmosis, TB, brucellosis, syphilis, poisoning with lead, carbon disulfide tetrachloroethane, leukaemia (CLL)) and with some drugs (e.g. aspirin, griseofulvin, haloperidol and phenytoin).
- A reduced lymphocyte count occurs in:
  - some infections
  - Hodgkin's disease
  - TB
  - post-irradiation
  - systemic lupus
  - renal failure
  - carcinomatosis
  - drugs (e.g. steroids, lithium and methysergide).

- Raised WBC and raised basophils are found in:
  - hypothyroidism
  - ulcerative colitis.
- Criteria for non-urgent referral to haematologists:
  - lymphocyte count of >10 × 10^9/l, and otherwise well.
- Criteria for urgent referral to haematologists:
  - lymphocytosis in association with:
    —Hb <10 g/dl or/and platelet <100 × 10^9/l
    —B symptoms
    —weight loss >10% in previous 6 months
    —severe night sweats
    —unexplained fever of >38°C for >2 weeks
  - lymphadenopathy
  - hepatomegaly or splenomegaly or both
  - extreme fatigue.
- A raised monocyte count (monocytosis) occurs in:
  - infectious mononucleosis
  - Hodgkin's disease
  - TB
  - subacute bacterial endocarditis
  - acute and chronic leukaemia
  - lymphoma
  - solid tumours
  - recovery after agranulocytosis.
- A lowered monocyte count may be found in:
  - chronic infection
  - treatment with glucocorticoids
  - infections producing endotoxins.

Morphological descriptions of neutrophils

- *Shift to the left*: the presence of immature granulocytes. It occurs as a reaction to pyogenic bacterial infection or after burns or haemorrhage.

- *Shift to the right (hypersegmented neutrophils)*: the appearance of neutrophils with >5 nuclear lobes. Characteristic of vitamin B_{12} or folate deficiency when accompanied by macrocytosis or renal failure, or as a congenital anomaly in the absence of macrocytosis.

- *Toxic granulation*: seen in infections and other toxic states, and is of no special significance.

- *Leucoerythroblastic anaemia*: occurs in severe infections, myeloproliferative disorders and in cases where infiltration of the bone marrow has occurred. A bone marrow biopsy is mandatory.

Large unstained cells

- This parameter is sometimes included in the automated differential WBC by some laboratories.

- Normal range (%):

  - adults, 0–6

  - children, 0–10.

- If *large unstained cells* are >6%, the laboratory will perform a manual differential count.

Pancytopenia

- All elements of cellular elements are reduced (red cells, white cells and platelets).

- It is due to bone marrow failure or premature destruction of the cells, and may be caused by:

  - malignant disease in the marrow

  - autoimmune disease (e.g. RA, SLE)

  - increased splenic activity or destruction (e.g. portal hypertension); aplastic anaemia, which can be due to drugs (e.g. antithyroids, antidepressants, anticoagulants, antibiotics, antihistamines, tranquillisers and thiazide diuretics)

- PA

- myelodysplastic syndrome

- acute leukaemia.

Monoclonal gammopathy of undetermined significance (MGUS)

- MGUS is a build-up of monoclonal antibodies (immunoglobulin), also called an M protein, produced by abnormal but non-cancerous plasma cells.

- Other causes of abnormal immunoglobulin production are:

  - multiple myeloma

  - Waldenstrom's macroglobulinaemia

  - primary amyloidosis

  - other lymphoproliferative disorders.

- In MGUS, the serum M protein is <3.0 g/dl and the bone marrow contains <10% plasma cells.

- MGUS occurs in

  - 3% of people over age 70 years

  - 6% of people over age 80 years

  - 14% of people over age 90 years.

- Transient monoclonal gammopathy can occur following some viral infections such as:

  - viral hepatitis and cytomegalovirus infection

  - cirrhosis

  - sarcoidosis

and also:

  - following bone marrow transplantation

  - in some cancers (colon, breast and prostate)

  - in autoimmune disorders (Sjögren's syndrome and RA)

  - following transplant surgery.

- Patients with MGUS are usually asymptomatic and discovered while being tested for other conditions.

- MGUS may progress to
  - multiple myeloma
  - macroglobulinaemia
  - amyloidosis plasmacytoma
  - malignant lymphoproliferative disorder.

- Baseline investigations should include FBC, serum calcium, creatinine and albumin, and serum protein electrophoresis and urine for total protein and Bence–Jones protein.

- When confirmed, requires annual review.

Myelodysplastic syndrome (MDS)

- This group of disorders is characterised by peripheral blood cytopenias and morphological abnormalities of the blood and marrow. It probably progresses to leukaemia.

- Five categories exist.

- Full blood count and film usually suggest MDS, showing cytopenia and dysplastic morphology. Macrocytosis and abnormal neutrophils are common. A marrow aspiration is required to confirm the diagnosis.

- It is most common in individuals over 50 years of age, unless there has been previous exposure to radio- or chemotherapy.

- Consider MDS in the elderly with refractory anaemia, bruising and occasionally recurrent infections, especially if cytopenia is present.

- Red cells, platelets and granulocytes may all be affected, or any combination or only one cell type may be involved (e.g. patients may present with a macrocytosis without the anaemia). In the absence of vitamin B_{12} or folate deficiency or hypothyroidism, pre-leukaemia may be suspected.

- A persistent monocytosis in the absence of TB or subacute bacterial endocarditis may be a precursor of pre-leukaemia.

- Bone marrow examination is required to make the diagnosis.

- Treatment is by transfusion; treat any infection.

- The expected survival period is 2 years, but it can range from 2–3 months to 10 years.

Special types of MDS
- *Sideroblastic anaemia*: white cells and platelets are normal; responds to pyridoxine and folate.

- *Chronic myelomonocytic leukaemia*: monocytosis and splenomegaly.

Chronic lymphatic leukaemia (CLL)

- Chronic lymphatic leukaemia is fairly common, particularly in the elderly.

- Presentation may be insidious, with an unexplained lymphocytosis.

- A lymphocyte count of $>15 \times 10^9/l$ requires referral to a haematologist for further investigation.

- In CLL there is often a normochromic normocytic anaemia.

- WCC may range from 50 to $200 \times 10^9/l$.

- Decreased platelets.

- There are five stages of CLL:

  - 0, lymphocytosis, normal marrow function except for increased lymphocytes

  - 1, lymphadenopathy in addition to the above

  - 2, splenomegaly plus lymphadenopathy or hepatomegaly

  - 3–4, either Hb <10 or platelets <100, indicating impaired bone marrow function.

- The prognosis is good for patients in stages 0–2 of the disease and poor for patients in stages 3 and 4 (about 2–3 years).

Drugs causing blood dyscrasias

- Idiosyncratic blood dyscrasias include neutropenia, thrombocytopenia and aplastic anaemia caused by a direct toxic effect on cell production by the drug or its metabolites.

- The incidence of blood dyscrasias increases with age of the patient, dose of the drug and duration of use of the drug. Renal or hepatic impairment and the concomitant use of other cytotoxic drugs will also increase the likelihood of reactions.

- Haemolytic anaemias may also occur when using penicillins, methyldopa, hydralazine, anti-malarials or sulphonamide antibiotics.

TABLE 1.1 Drugs causing blood dyscrasias

Neutropenia	Thrombocytopenia	Aplastic anaemia
Captopril	Heparin	NSAIDs
Phenothiazines	Anticonvulsants	Anticonvulsants
Carbimazole	Gold	Gold
Sulphonamides	Sulphonamides	Sulphonamides
Clozapine	Rifampicin	Chloramphenicol
Mianserin	Quinine/quinidine	Penicillamine
Propylthiouracil		Phenothiazines

PLATELETS

- Normal range ($\times 10^9$/l) is 150–400.

Abnormal test results
Low platelet count of $<100 \times 10^9$/l should be repeated in a bottle containing citrate, not ethylenediaminetetra-acetic acid (EDTA).
- Low platelet counts are found in:
  - bone marrow hypoplasia/aplasia
  - bone marrow infiltration
  - vitamin B_{12}/folate deficiency/iron deficiency
  - immune thrombocytopenia, including drugs (e.g. thiazides, gold and sulphonamides)
  - infections
  - hypersplenism
  - DIC
  - ITP
  - severe infections following massive haemorrhage

- liver disease/alcohol

- uraemia

- patients who have received many blood transfusions.

- Platelet count less than 50 requires immediate discussion with haematologist.

- Increased platelet counts should be repeated together with ESR, CRP, and autoantibodies, and may be found in:

  - trauma

  - infection and inflammation (e.g. chronic inflammatory bowel disease)

  - malignancy and myeloproliferative disorders (e.g. myelofibrosis, essential thrombocythaemia, chronic leukaemia)

  - rebound thrombocytosis, which occurs after haemorrhage, haemolysis and post-splenectomy

  - post-exercise.

- Giant platelets may be seen in a blood film, and may occur following any acute illness or haemorrhage. They may also precede some forms of leukaemia. In an otherwise healthy person with this finding, the test should be repeated in 4–6 weeks.

BLOOD COAGULATION TESTS

- A family and drug history is essential, and the following clotting and bleeding time tests may be of help.

- Acquired clotting defects are more common than congenital ones.

- In patients who present with bruising or frank bleeding, clotting disorders should be considered.

- Purpura, which is characterised by flat, sharp-edged, dark red lesions which do not blanch on pressure, may be caused by thrombocytopenia or increased vascular fragility, as in senile purpura or patients on long-term steroid therapy, or with Cushing's disease.

- About 70% of patients who present with bruising will have no haematological abnormality.

- Anticoagulation therapy is the commonest cause of acquired bleeding disorders. Warfarin therapy affects factors II, VII, IX and X.

- Liver disease can also cause abnormal bleeding via a number of mechanisms.

- Of the inherited disorders associated with abnormal bleeding, haemophilia (which includes haemophilia A (due to factor VIII deficiency), and haemophilia B (due to factor IX deficiency, and also known as Christmas disease) is the commonest.

- Infiltrative disease of the bone marrow, seen in aplastic anaemia, leukaemia and malignant disease, can produce thrombocytopenia, which may also be caused by some drugs, such as thiazide diuretics, quinine, quinidine, methyldopa, digoxin, and some infections (e.g. rubella, glandular fever and mumps).

- Acute idiopathic thrombocytopenic purpura is most commonly seen 2–3 weeks after an upper respiratory infection. In children, especially boys, Henoch–Schönlein purpura may present with a rash, most commonly distributed on the extensor surfaces and buttocks, accompanied by fever, myalgia, joint pains, abdominal pain and glomerulonephritis.

- Acute idiopathic thrombocytopenic purpura will present 5–10 times in the average GP's career.

- Vascular causes of purpura include senile purpura, cough purpura in children with whooping cough, and rare connective tissue disorders.

Plasma fibrinogen
- Normal range (g/l) is 1.5–4.0 (0.2–0.4%).

Abnormal test results
- Decreased levels are found in:
  - liver disease
  - DIC.

- Increased levels are found:
  - following tissue damage or infection
  - in pregnancy

- in nephrotic syndrome

- in collagen disease.

- Patients with high plasma fibrinogen levels (>3.5 g/l) as well as high serum cholesterol (>6.2 mmol/l) and a systolic blood pressure of >140 mmHg have a twelvefold higher incidence of heart attack than do those with a fibrinogen level of <2.9 g/l. Reducing weight and cholesterol, as well as stopping smoking, lowers fibrinogen – as do clofibrate and bezafibrate.

Fibrin degradation products
- Normal range (mg/l) is <10.

Abnormal test results
- Raised levels are found in:

  - increased fibrinolysis such as post-MI, deep vein thrombosis (DVT), pulmonary embolism (PE) and DIC

  - liver or renal failure (secondary to DIC).

Activated partial thromboplastin time
- Also known as kaolin cephalin clotting time (KCCT).

- Normal range is 26–39 seconds: laboratory reference >40 ± 7 is abnormal and always requires investigation.

- A measurement of the intrinsic side of the clotting factor cascade.

- This is the most suitable test for monitoring IV heparin, but not subcutaneously.

- APTT, normal range 1.5–2.5 for someone on heparin therapy.

Abnormal test results
- Prolonged KCCT occurs in the following:

  - heparin therapy

  - clotting factor deficiency syndromes (usually factors VIII and IX, and occasionally factors XI and XII, e.g. Von Willebrand's disease)

- presence of clotting inhibiting factors, such as may be present in the para-proteinaemias or lupus

- liver disease

- after massive transfusions.

Prothrombin time

- This is one of the tests used to monitor oral anticoagulants.

- Normal range (seconds) is control ±4 (usually 13–15).

- It tests the extrinsic clotting system (factors II, VII and X).

- The result is inversely proportional to the prothrombin content of the blood tested.

INR

See next section, 'Warfarin in practice'.

- The INR is the ratio of the patient's prothrombin time (the time taken for plasma to form a fibrin clot when mixed with tissue thromboplastin) and the control prothrombin time raised to the power of the International Sensitivity Index.

- An INR of 1 represents the clotting time of an individual with normal clotting. An INR of 2 indicates that the sample of blood takes twice as long to clot.

Thrombo test

- This is used in some centres to measure warfarin therapy.

- Normal range (%) is 7–17.

WARFARIN IN PRACTICE

Warfarin antagonises vitamin K, leading to depletion of several clotting factors and the inhibition of thrombin formation. The full anticoagulant effect takes 24–48 hours to develop, so heparin must be given concurrently if an immediate effect is required. Warfarin is commonly used in the prevention and treatment of venous thromboembolism; the prevention of embolism from a mechanical heart valve prosthesis, or in the presence of atrial fibrillation complicating rheumatic valvular disease and, increasingly, in patients with non-rheumatic atrial fibrillation.

Control

The warfarin dosage is adjusted according to the INR, which should be measured before warfarin is started. The recommended starting dose in acute situations is 10 mg daily for 2 days, and less for those with heart failure, the very elderly and patients with impaired liver function. Initially, the INR should be measured on alternate days, with progressive lengthening of the interval as control is established. *The interval between tests should never exceed 8 weeks.* In non-urgent situations (e.g. the presence of non-rheumatic atrial fibrillation), a more gradual introduction of warfarin at a dose of 4 mg daily may be preferable and reduces the required frequency of INR tests. The maintenance dose of warfarin is best taken at the same time each day.

The commonest cause of unexpected test results is non-compliance with the recommended warfarin dosage. *For the prophylaxis of DVT, including surgery on high-risk patients, a target range of 2.0–2.5 is advised.*

In the treatment of DVT or PE the target INR is 2–3, and in the presence of a mechanical heart valve prosthesis, the INR target range is 3.0–4.5.

In the case of some bileaflet valve prostheses, particularly in the aortic position, some authorities recommend a target INR in the lower part of this range, i.e. 2–3, but not below.

Studies among patients with non-rheumatic atrial fibrillation suggest that a target INR of 2.0 may be sufficient to provide protection against stroke. In the presence of previous cerebral ischaemia, a target ratio of 2.0–3.9 has been advised.

Important drug interactions

A large number of drugs can either potentiate or antagonise the anticoagulant effect of warfarin by interfering with absorption or metabolism either of the drug or of vitamin K.

Drugs that are likely to potentiate the anticoagulant effect of warfarin

These include alcohol, aspirin, non-steroidal anti-inflammatory drugs (NSAIDs), steroids, amiodarone, propafenone, some antibiotics (ciprofloxacin, co-trimoxazole, sulphonamides, erythromycin, amino glycosides, metronidazole and possibly ampicillin), fibrates, simvastatin, thyroxine, dextropropoxyphene, dipyridamole, miconazole, ketoconazole, allopurinol, cimetidine, danazol and some antidepressants.

Drugs that are likely to antagonise the anticoagulant effect of warfarin

These include oral contraceptives, some anti-epileptics (carbamazepine and primidone, phenytoin), griseofulvin and rifampicin.

In addition, *major dietary changes can influence the anticoagulant effect of warfarin*, such as a substantial increase in alcohol (which enhances the effect) or in vegetable consumption (which antagonises it). When in doubt (e.g. during a prolonged course of treatment involving antibiotics or a NSAID), or if there is a substantial change in the patient's health (particularly an increase in heart failure or a febrile illness), it is important to increase the frequency of INR checks.

Dentistry

Dental surgery may be undertaken in most patients with little risk of haemorrhage if the INR is ≤2.0. More major surgery requires that the relative risks of stopping warfarin or continuing with anticoagulants throughout the operative period be assessed on an individual patient basis by the specialist team concerned.

Pregnancy

Warfarin crosses the placenta and between weeks 6 and 9 it is teratogenic (nasal hypoplasia – stippled epiphyses). It may also cause foetal haemorrhage, particularly in the third trimester. None the less, maintenance of warfarin therapy may represent the safest option in some circumstances (e.g. pregnant women with diseased or prosthetic heart valves).

Heparin may be given subcutaneously and does not cross the placenta. It may cause thrombocytopenia and osteoporosis if given for more than 6 months.

Duration of treatment with warfarin

Up to 12 months

- Prophylaxis of DVT, including high-risk surgery.

- Treatment of an established venous thrombosis.

- Treatment of an established pulmonary embolus.

- MI, anterior myocardial infarct (usually a minimum of 3 months of treatment with warfarin).

- Xenograft heart valve replacement.

- Coronary artery bypass-graft.

Lifelong treatment with warfarin

- Recurrent venous thromboembolism.

- Embolic complications of rheumatic heart disease and atrial fibrillation.

- Cardiac prosthetic valve replacement and arterial grafts.

THROMBOPHILIA

- This is an inherited or acquired tendency towards abnormal clotting.

- It is two to three times more common than bleeding disorders.

- Consider thrombophilia in people under 40 years of age with recurrent thromboembolic disease or a primary thromboembolic event with a strong family history (*see* antiphospholipid syndrome, p. 38).

- Check antithrombin III, protein C and protein S, lupus anticoagulant and anticardiolipin antibodies, as well as disorders of fibrinolysis.

- A positive family history may be present, and should lead to screening of other at-risk relatives.

- Other predisposing factors for thrombosis coexist in 50% of cases.

- Refer the patient to a haematologist.

NB: Thrombophilic patients who suffer thrombotic episodes will need long-term prophylaxis with warfarin.

Management of patients with thrombophilia

Patients who have a tendency to thrombosis have it because they have a disorder of the blood (e.g. a coagulation defect or a cellular abnormality such as polycythaemia) or a defect of the vessel wall. Where enhanced coagulation is the primary cause, the disorder is referred to as *thrombophilia*.

In patients with thrombophilia, the mechanisms that normally inhibit thrombosis are impaired, resulting, for example, in thrombosis at an early age or recurrent thrombosis. The risk of thrombosis is increased by obesity, immobility, trauma, pregnancy and malignancy. Thrombophilia may be inherited or acquired.

Inherited thrombophilia

Inherited resistance to activated protein C2 and inherited deficiencies of antithrombin III, protein C and protein S predispose to thrombosis. Inherited resistance to activated protein C occurs in up to 7% of the population and produces a variant factor V (factor V Leiden) which, when detected in women, can indicate a predisposition to thrombosis during pregnancy and while taking the oral contraceptive pill.

Acquired thrombophilia

The most frequent cause of acquired thrombophilia is the antiphos pholipid syndrome, which is caused by the presence of lupus anticoagulant and/or anticardiolipin antibody predisposing to venous and arterial thrombosis.

Who should be investigated?

The following observations should alert the physician to the possibility of thrombophilia:
- venous thromboembolism in a patient aged under 40 years
- recurrent venous thrombosis or thrombophlebitis
- venous thrombosis in an unusual site (e.g. mesenteric or cerebral vein)
- skin necrosis, especially in a patient taking warfarin
- arterial thrombosis in a patient aged under 30 years
- a family history of venous thromboembolism
- recurrent foetal loss
- unexplained neonatal thrombosis.

Investigations

These should include the following:
- full blood count, including platelet count
- prothrombin time (*see* p. 33)
- activated partial thromboplastin time (*see* p. 32)
- thrombin time
- reptilase time
- fibrinogen concentration (*see* p. 31)

- plasma antithrombin III activity (82–120 IU/dl)

- plasma C function estimate (70–140 IU/dl)

- plasma free protein S level (54–123 IU/dl)

- plasma APC-R (the screening test for factor V Leiden) (2.61–3.45)

- lupus anticoagulant screen.

Antiphospholipid syndrome (Hughes' syndrome)

- Antiphospholipid syndrome may be suspected when a patient has suffered from venous thrombosis, or thrombophlebitis, arterial thrombosis or recurrent miscarriage AND has antiphospholipid antibodies.

- Antiphospholipid antibodies comprise:

  - anticardialipin antibodies

  - beta glycoprotein antibodies.

- Antiphospholipid antibodies:

  - <10 U G phospholipid (GPL)/ml   absence of antibodies
  - 10–25 U GPL/ml   low titre, confirm with a further new sample
  - >25 U GPL/ml   significant titre.

- As well as antiphospholipid antibodies, clotting studies are performed looking for lupus anticoagulant. Lupus anticoagulant is likely to be present if the activated partial thromboplastin time (previously known as the kaolin cephalin clotting time or KCCT) is prolonged (abnormal >40 ± 7 seconds) (*see* p. 32).

- Antiphospholipid antibodies should be requested in the case of:

  - young patients with unexpected DVT

  - young patients with unexpected MI or cerebrovascular accident

  - all patients with SLE

  - patients with recurrent headaches, especially recurrent migraine.

- Female patients with antiphospholipid syndrome can be treated with aspirin or heparin and this dramatically reduces the risk of recurrent miscarriage.

HAEMOGLOBINOPATHIES

Because many inherited Hb and red cell enzyme disorders confer partial protection against malaria, haemoglobinopathies are more common in ethnic groups that originate from endemic malaria zones. In the UK, patients of Afro-Caribbean, Asian and Mediterranean origin are more likely to carry the genetic disorders.

Hb electrophoresis

Hb A2 level	normal	1.5–3.5%
Hb F	normal	<1%

Sickle-cell disease

- Haemolysis may lead to anaemia and increased folic acid requirements.

- It mainly affects people of African, Afro-Caribbean, Middle Eastern and Mediterranean descent.

- About 5,000 people are affected in the UK, with many more having the sickle-cell trait.

- The clinical syndromes have variable penetration, and some individuals are more affected than others.

- Infants born with sickle-cell disease are at high risk of death due to overwhelming pneumococcal infection. Symptoms are rarely present during the first 6 months of life, due to the presence of foetal Hb, but often appear during the first 2 years of life, as foetal Hb levels decrease. The affected infant suffers from recurrent respiratory infections, failure to thrive and anaemia. Chronic haemolysis leads to anaemia (Hb is often around 8 g/dl, with 10–30% reticulocytes). Pulmonary complications, stroke and meningitis are common causes of death.

- The diagnosis is made by electrophoresis.

- Other children and adults often present with pain 'crises', such as repeated episodes of asymmetrical joint or bone pain, sometimes associated with abdominal or chest pain.

Thalassaemia

- This is the most common haemoglobinopathy, affecting 4% of the world's population and 5% of the population of England and Wales.

- It is the most common inherited disease in the UK among immigrants from the Mediterranean, East Africa, Asia (including South East Asia and Vietnam) and the Caribbean.

- Two forms exist, depending on which globin chain is affected (alpha or beta). Beta-thalassaemia can be divided into major (found in those who have the disease) and minor (found in those who carry the disease).

- Thalassaemia confers protection against *Plasmodium falciparum* (malaria).

Beta-thalassaemia major

- It begins in early childhood.

- Severe anaemia leads to frequent blood transfusions.

- Splenomegaly occurs.

- Tissue hypoxia, iatrogenic iron overload resulting in liver damage, cardiac failure and endocrine failure usually result in death before the age of 30 years.

- Patients should receive regular iron chelation therapy with subcutaneous desferrioxamine.

Thalassaemia minor (the carrier state)

- This is asymptomatic, although it may be suspected when a blood film shows a microcytic hypochromic anaemia with target cells, poikilocytosis and basophil stippling, together with a normal serum ferritin (unlike iron deficiency, where the ferritin would also be lowered).

- The importance of thalassaemia minor is in the prevention of the homozygous thalassaemia major.

- Hb is often 10–15 g/dl, while RBC is higher, and MCH and MCHC are lower than in comparable cases of iron-deficiency anaemia.

Alpha-thalassaemia

- This is distinguished from beta-thalassaemia by electrophoresis.

Glucose-6-phosphate dehydrogenase deficiency
Most common cause of haemolytic anaemia

This affects ethnic groups similar to those affected by thalassaemia and can lead to severe haemolytic disease. The gene is carried on the X-chromosome, so usually only males are affected. The Mediterranean type may lead to *favism*, namely acute intravascular haemolysis following the ingestion of certain types of bean.

Glucose-6-phosphate dehydrogenase deficiency renders affected individuals susceptible to haemolysis produced by certain oxidant drugs and infections.

Laboratory findings

- Haemoglobinopathies and glucose-6-phosphate dehydrogenase deficiency often show a microcytic anaemia.

- In the thalassaemia trait there are often a low MCV and MCHC and high red cell count.

- Target cells may be seen.

- Electrophoresis is diagnostic.

B-type natriuretic peptide (BNP)

- Normal values: age/sex range available from local laboratory.

  - BNP <100 pg/ml suggests heart failure is unlikely.

  - BNP >400 pg/ml suggests that heart failure is likely.

- BNP is a peptide present in the blood that is derived from cardiac pro-BNP and is released by the ventricles in heart failure.

- Before requesting BNP, a 12-lead ECG should be performed which is likely to show one of six abnormalities in the presence of heart failure:

  - Q waves

  - left ventricular hypertrophy

  - atrial fibrillation

  - left bundle branch block

  - poor R wave progression

  - left axis deviation.

- *See* Figure 1.1 for the management of suspected heart failure.

- False-positive BNP results may occur with ischaemic heart disease, left ventricular hypertrophy, CKD, chronic obstructive pulmonary disease, tachycardia, diabetes and cirrhosis.

- False-negative results may occur in patients being treated with cardiovascular drugs, e.g. diuretics, angiotensin-converting enzyme inhibitors, angiotensin receptor blockers and beta-blockers.

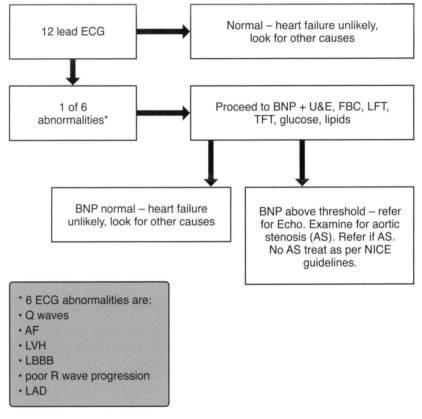

FIGURE 1.1 Suspected heart failure because of history, symptoms and signs

D-dimers

- Normal value <190 µg/l.

- Elevated D-dimers are found in clinical conditions such as:

  - DVT

  - PE

- DIC
- trauma.
- D-dimers are sensitive markers for the above conditions occurring in the previous week.
- D-dimers should not be used alone to confirm venous thromboembolism, which usually requires ultrasonography and/or VQ scan, or pulmonary arteriography.
- Raised levels can also be found in:
  - pregnancy
  - age over 70 years
  - post-operative patients
  - inflammation
  - infection
  - cancer
  - renal failure.

COMMON HAEMATOLOGICAL TERMS
Anisocytes (red cells of variable size)
- Abnormally shaped cells that are sometimes associated with megaloblastic anaemia, partially treated iron deficiency and some conditions in which the anaemia is secondary to systemic disease.

Poikilocytosis (red cells of variable shape)
- Tear-shaped cells suggestive of an erythropoiesis defect that are seen in megaloblastic anaemias and myelofibrosis.

Spherocytes
- Abnormally thick red cells that are associated with:
  - hereditary spherocytosis
  - haemolytic disorders
  - severe burns
  - *Clostridium welchii* septicaemia.

Eliptocytes

- Pencil-shaped cells that are seen in:
  - iron-deficiency anaemia
  - mild congenital haemolytic anaemia.

Target cells

- Cells that are associated with:
  - iron-deficiency anaemia
  - haemoglobinopathy (including thalassaemia, liver disorders and splenectomy).

Spur cells

- Cells that are seen in severe hepatic disease.

Burr cells

- Irregularly contracted red cells that are seen in renal disease.

Fragmented red cells

- Cells that are seen:
  - in DIC
  - post-splenectomy
  - in patients with a heart valve prosthesis.

Crenation

- Curly- or wavy-edged red cells – sometimes indicative of renal disease. Therefore urea and electrolytes are appropriate as the next investigation.
- Crenation occurs:
  - in hypothyroidism
  - as an artefact
  - in the elderly.

Hypochromasia

- The condition in which cells take stain less readily/intensely than usual.

- It is a feature of:
  - iron deficiency
  - thalassaemia
  - lead poisoning.

Polychromasia

- Red cells staining slightly blue, associated with an increased number of reticulocytes.

- It *always implies pathology*, and is found in:
  - haemolytic anaemia
  - haemorrhage
  - response to haematinics
  - marrow infiltration
  - severe hypoxia.

Dimorphic red cells

- These may be a feature of sideroblastic anaemia and may also be seen in patients being treated for anaemia secondary to haematinics deficiency, and in patients post transfusion.

Anisocytosis

- Variation in the size of red cells.

Echinocytes

- Multiple spicules on the red-cell surface, usually associated with mild haemolysis.

Acanthocytes

- Irregularly contracted red cells, seen in liver disease.

Rouleaux

- Stacks of red cells in the blood film reflected by an increase in the ESR.

- They may be present in:

  - acute infections

  - conditions where abnormal plasma proteins are present (e.g. myeloma).

EDTA changes

- Potassium (K^+) EDTA is the anticoagulant of choice for blood counting and enables some of the elements of the blood, especially the platelets, to remain stable for several days.

- The Hb content of a sample does not vary with time even if haemolysis occurs.

- Some changes occur in the white cells (in particular, neutrophils disintegrate), hence the total WBC will be affected and an apparent neutropenia or lymphocytosis may occur.

Heinz bodies

- These may be found in haemolytic states, especially when drug induced.

Pancytopenia

- This may be due to:

  - bone marrow failure

  - premature destruction of cells

  - malignant disease

  - haematological and non-haematological disease (e.g. RA, SLE, myelodysplasia, PA)

  - increased splenic activity or destruction (e.g. portal hypertension)

  - aplastic anaemia, which can be due to drugs (e.g. antithyroids, antidepressants, antibiotics, antihistamines, tranquillisers, thiazide diuretics).

Chapter 2

Microbiology

GASTROINTESTINAL ORGANISMS

- Examination for ova, cysts and parasites is usually performed routinely.

- All infectious diarrhoea is notifiable as dysentery or food poisoning to the Consultant in Communicable Disease Control in order to locate and eradicate the source.

- Stool specimens should be sent to the laboratory in a sterile, screw-cap container. More than one specimen may be helpful in the identification of organisms such as *Giardia lamblia*.

- Transport the specimen to the laboratory as soon as possible.

- An appropriate plastic container should be used so that dehydration of the specimen is avoided.

- Stool specimens that are to be examined for mobile trophozoites should be kept at room temperature and examined shortly after collection, while the organisms are still active.

- Examination of faeces for ova or cysts can be done on a 'cold' specimen.

Food poisoning

- The organisms most commonly found are those of the salmonella group, such as *Salmonella typhimurium* and *Salmonella enteritidis.*

- Food poisoning is also commonly caused by *Staphylococcus aureus* and *Bacillus cereus*, which produce an exotoxin. Occasionally, *Clostridium perfringens* and, rarely, *Clostridium botulinum* may be the causative organisms.

- The following should be sent to the laboratory in suspected cases:

  - portion of food suspected

  - stools as soon as these have been passed.

Salmonella

Transmission

- This is mainly from food (raw meat, poultry and eggs); rarely from person to person.

Presentation

- Diarrhoea predominates; abdominal pain, vomiting and fever may occur.

Treatment

- Ill or toxic patients require admission to an infectious diseases hospital.

- Patients usually require supportive treatment only, i.e. fluids.

  NB: Treatment with certain antibiotics can limit the duration of excretion and may be required in severe cases.

Shigella

- Stool samples should be delivered fresh to the laboratory.

Transmission

- This occurs via flies, fingers, food and faeces.

Presentation
- The same symptoms as are caused by *Salmonella* (diarrhoea predominates).
- Common in young children (<8 years), particularly those attending junior schools and nurseries.
- Occasionally the patient may become unwell or toxic.

Treatment
- If the patient is unwell, symptomatic treatment should be given.
- Exclude infected children from school until the diarrhoea has resolved.
- Septrin is rarely indicated.

Giardia lamblia (*Giardia intestinalis*)
- Three stool specimens may be required at 24-hour intervals, as cysts are only excreted intermittently.

Transmission
- This is mainly via contaminated water or faeco-oral spread. The organism may be found in stools, especially if the patient has recently returned from abroad having contracted persistent diarrhoea.
- Spread may be rapid in nurseries and junior schools, where faeco-oral spread predominates.

Presentation
- Fatty, offensive and persistent diarrhoea (malabsorption type).

Treatment
- Flagyl daily for 3 days:
  - adult, 2 g
  - child, 7–10 years, 1 g
  - child, 3–7 years, 600 mg.

Investigating adults with diarrhoea

- If a patient has diarrhoea that persists for more than 48–72 hours, then sending a stool culture for microbiological investigation may be useful.

- Unformed stools will be routinely tested for:

  - *Salmonella*

  - *Shigella*

  - *Campylobacter*

  - *Escherichia coli* O157

  - *Cryptosporidium*

  - *C. difficile* if patient is over 65 years.

Recent travel abroad

- The laboratory will not usually process requests for ova, cysts and parasites unless the patient has travelled abroad and this is stated on the request form.

- Indicating the country travelled to and from is useful.

Treating adults with diarrhoea

- Treatment with antibiotics for patients with diarrhoea is rarely required, except sometimes in cases of:

  - campylobacter (which can be treated with erythromycin) or

  - patients with *Clostridium difficile*, which can be treated with metronidazole 400 mg tds for 10 days. During the course of treatment the patient may improve and diarrhoea may resolve or diarrhoea may recur. Whatever the outcome, treatment should still continue for the full 10-day period. At the end of the treatment period, if the patient still has diarrhoea or blood in the stools or abdominal pain, then advice from the local microbiologist should be sought.

Clostridium difficile

- Consider *Clostridium difficile* infection in patients with persistent diarrhoea if they are under age 65 years and have risk factors for *Clostridium difficile* such as:

- having been discharged from hospital within the previous 3 months

- residence in a nursing or residential home

- having had antibiotics prescribed within the previous month.

- If *Clostridium difficile* is suspected, request stool examination for *Clostridium difficile* toxin.

- Over-prescribing proton pump inhibitors may be associated with increased incidence of infection with *Clostridium difficile.*

- For treatment discuss with microbiology department, usually metronidazole 400 mg tds for a full 10 days, whether the diarrhoea resolves or not.

Schistosomiasis

- Worms take 6–10 weeks before producing eggs, so testing the stool for ova should not be done until 12 weeks after exposure.

- Serological testing (enzyme-linked immunosorbent assay) is usually positive and is a more sensitive test than stool testing.

Vibrio cholerae

- This requires a special culture medium and will not be looked for by laboratories unless there is a history of travel to an endemic area (usually the tropics).

Transmission

- This is via water or food contaminated with sewage, the unclean hands of a person with cholera, or by flies. Person-to-person transmission is rare.

Presentation

- Profuse watery diarrhoea and occasionally vomiting. Dehydration may lead to collapse.

Campylobacter jejuni

- The most common cause of bacterial diarrhoea.

- Requires 48 hours' incubation.

Transmission
- Unpasteurised milk and stream water are often implicated, but it is quite common for the source to remain unidentified.

- Campylobacter is found in the gut and carcass of chickens and other animals, and can be spread during their preparation.

- Person-to-person transmission is rare.

Presentation
- Abdominal pain (sometimes severe abdominal cramps), diarrhoea and feeling generally unwell for up to 2 weeks. Vomiting is uncommon.

Treatment
- Rarely requires treatment.

- Erythromycin may be used, especially if the patient is immunosuppressed or there are severe abdominal cramps.

Helicobacter pylori
- This is associated with chronic gastritis and relapsing duodenal ulcers. It cannot be isolated from stool culture, but can be grown from gastric biopsy at endoscopy or its presence deduced from a radioisotope carbon dioxide breath test. An exhaled breath test with a value of <0.25 suggests that no *H. pylori* is present, whereas a value of >0.25 suggests that *Helicobacter* is present.

- Can be eradicated with Flagyl, amoxycillin and a proton pump inhibitor.

- The treatment of proven cases of known peptic ulceration remains controversial.

Cryptosporidium (parvum)
- This protozoan is common in animal faeces.

- Sometimes seen in young children who have contact with young animals (e.g. on school trips to a farm or in contaminated mains water supplies).

Transmission
- This is via infected cattle, milk or water (especially swimming pools).

Presentation
- Self-limiting gastroenteritis in normal individuals, or it may even be asymptomatic.
- Life-threatening diarrhoea in immunologically depressed individuals.

Treatment
- No effective treatment is available.
- The infection is usually self-limiting, but in immunocompromised patients (e.g. those with AIDS) it may be life-threatening.

Enteropathogenic *Escherichia coli*
- This is detectable using specific agglutination tests.

Viral causes of gastroenteritis
- These can be identified using an electron microscope, or enzyme-linked immunosorbent assay if available. Rotavirus and small round viruses are the most commonly detected organisms.

Enterobius vermicularis (pinworm, threadworm or seatworm)
- Diagnosis is best made with a sticky tape slide collecting eggs at the perianal margin.

Treatment
- Piperazine:
    - 6 years to adult, 1 sachet
    - 1–5 years, $^2/_3$ sachet
    - 3 months to 1 year, $^1/_3$ sachet.
- Repeat after 14 days.
- The whole family should be treated as well as the affected individual.

- It is important to cut and scrub fingernails and to change underclothing and bed linen.

Listeriosis

Transmission

- This is via contaminated food, especially soft cheese, unpasteurised dairy products, chicken and pre-packed salads.

- The organism can grow at refrigeration temperatures (4°C).

Presentation

- Infection is mainly seen in the very young, the very old, pregnant women and the immunocompromised.

- In healthy people, the illness resembles a mild influenza and the diagnosis is rarely made.

- In pregnant women, it may affect the foetus and can lead to miscarriage, stillbirth or severe illness in the newborn infant.

  NB: A definitive microbiological diagnosis of listeriosis in pregnancy can only be made from a blood culture. Check with the laboratory to ensure that the correct culture is used. Blood cultures should be sent to the laboratory as soon as possible and should not be refrigerated.

Procedure

- It is very important that any request form accompanying samples from a patient in whom listeriosis is suspected should state this fact clearly. Clinical samples may not be routinely examined for *Listeria*.

Treatment

- A variety of antibiotics (including ampicillin, erythromycin and tetracycline) is used to treat listeriosis.

Investigations that can help diagnose travel-related infections

- Blood:

  - full blood count with differential white cell count and thick and thin blood films for malarial parasites

- erythrocyte sedimentation rate and C-reactive protein
- liver function tests
- viral serology including hepatitis serology.

- Urine:
  - mid-stream urine specimen (MSU) and request examination for ova, cysts and parasites if schistosomiasis is suspected.

- Faeces:
  - for ova, cysts and parasites.

Extended spectrum beta-lactamase (ESBL) producers, Amp C beta-lactamase (Amp-C) producers and vancomycin-resistant *Enterococci* guidelines

- ESBL and Amp-C producers are multi-resistant Gram-negative (usually bowel) bacteria. These are resistant to several commonly used antibiotics such as cefuroxime, gentamicin and ciprofloxacin. The resistances vary between each isolate.

- Vancomycin-resistant *Enterococci* are Gram-positive bacteria, resistant to both vancomycin and teicoplanin to varying degrees. They may also be resistant to ampicillin and gentamicin.

- Most antibiotic-resistant bacteria originate in hospitals and are spread into the community. Vancomycin-resistant *Enterococci* are an interesting exception to this and can originate in the community as well as in hospitals, possibly from colonised farm animals via contaminated meat.

- These bacteria can live in the bowel and be excreted in the faeces. Patients may carry these bacteria for many months.

- ESBL or Amp-C producers are passed from person to person, either directly or indirectly, via faecal contamination of hands and objects and then introduced into the mouth (faeco-oral spread). These patients may not be ill, but are colonised with these antibiotic-resistant bacteria, and can potentially spread them to susceptible patients.

- Other sites that can be colonised include:
  - urinary catheters

- chronic wounds and ulcers

- the throat and mouth.

- Currently this type of contamination is being found most often in the long-term care setting such as nursing homes and residential homes. The problem is often first identified, however, when an MSU is submitted to the microbiology lab for culture.

- The bacteria can survive on the hands and in the environment, e.g. door handles and telephones, for between 4 and 8 hours, so it can be readily spread around the patients' and healthcare workers' environment by touching. For this reason, killing the bacteria, with the alcohol hand rub placed at the end of every patient's bed, is vitally important.

- Other control measures in a nursing or care home should be discussed with the local microbiology department.

  - The Infection Control Team must be informed on diagnosis or readmission.

  - A dedicated toilet or commode must be used in all cases.

  - Special attention should be placed on using gloves, aprons and decontaminating hands with alcohol hand rub.

  - Screening may be undertaken at the discretion of the Infection Control Team.

Infections with ESBL and Amp-C producers

- Patients with urinary catheters will remain colonised while the catheter is in place.

- Patients with non-healing wounds such as pressure sores and leg ulcers will remain colonised until these wounds heal.

- Patients without urinary catheters and wounds/ulcers may remain colonised in the faeces and urine for many months.

Prevention of transmission with ESBL and Amp-C producers

- Hand washing for the healthcare worker and the patient before the patient eats or receives oral medications. If alcohol hand rub is available, the healthcare worker should use this.

UROGENITAL ORGANISMS

NB: Swabs must be taken from appropriate sites, e.g. vaginal for-nices or endocervical, and appropriately labelled and sent in the correct culture medium.

The high vaginal swab (HVS) is not good at detecting gonococcus but may detect trichomonas, candida and bacterial vaginosis. At room temperature a HVS will keep for 24 hours before culture, but it will be unsuitable for testing for gonococci after 12 hours.

• Many different organisms may be present at the same time.

• Refer to genito-urinary clinic for most appropriate investigations and contact tracing.

• Culture of some organisms is difficult, and a specific culture medium must be used.

• In cases of suspected pelvic inflammatory disease, an endocervical swab should be taken for *Neisseria gonorrhoeae* (only a 40% detection rate) and placed in the correct medium, and a further swab taken for *Chlamydia* in the chlamydia transport medium.

• In men, a cotton-tipped wire swab should be taken from 3–4 cm inside the urethra and sent to the laboratory in a transport medium.

Herpes genitalis
• This is a common cause of genital ulceration.

Presentation
• In men, an erythematous red area develops, usually on the prepuce, followed by vesicles.

• In women, the most common sites of vesicles are the labia majora and minora, cervix and perineum.

Diagnosis
• This is confirmed by sending material from the ulcer in virus transport medium for culture, although herpes will survive in Stuart's transport medium.

• Differential diagnosis includes:
  • primary chancre of syphilis

- secondary infection after scratching

- scabies

- lesions and trauma secondary to sexual intercourse.

Treatment
- Analgesics for pain relief.

- Zovirax cream 5% and oral Zovirax 200 mg × 5 od for 5 days.

- In frequently recurrent herpes, prophylaxis with oral Zovirax 200 mg 1–4 times daily.

Gonorrhoea
- About 60% of affected women are asymptomatic.

- Dysuria in a young man with a normal urinary tract is more likely to be due to urethritis than to urinary tract infection (UTI).

Presentation
- In men, there is discomfort in the urethra followed by a creamy, thick, yellow-green, purulent discharge.

- In women, there is a vaginal discharge, dysuria, frequency of micturition, backache or abdominal pain.

- *Trichomonas* is also present in 50% of positive cases.

Diagnosis
- In men, a swab of urethral discharge should be sent for staining, microscopic examination and culture.

- In women, swabs from the urethra and cervix should be sent for culture.

- Swabs should be transported in Stuart's medium in a bottle with a screw top, or as charcoal swabs.

Treatment
- Seek advice from a genito-urinary clinic with regard to further treatment and contact tracing.

- A single dose of 2.4 mega-units of procaine penicillin, or 3 g ampicillin or 3 g amoxycillin in a single dose, each with probenecid 2 g orally, should be given.

- For patients who are allergic to penicillin, or in cases where there is a high incidence (>5%) of penicillinase-producing *N. gonorrhoeae*, treat with spectinomycin, 2 g intramuscularly, or kanamycin, 2 g intramuscularly.

- Single-dose ciprofloxacin may be effective.

Trichomonas vaginalis

- This is a microscopic parasite.

- It may be an incidental finding on a cervical smear.

- It may occur in association with other venereal diseases.

- Infection may be asymptomatic.

Presentation

- In men, the urethra or its extensions may be infected and cause reinfection of the partner.

- In women, there is a frothy vaginal discharge with vaginal tenderness, swollen and inflamed vulva, and pain on urination.

Diagnosis

- A diagnosis must be made before any treatment is given.

- Mix discharge from the vagina with warm saline solution and examine under the microscope to detect parasites.

- *T. vaginalis* can be cultured.

Treatment

- If symptomatic, give Flagyl 200 mg tds × 1 week or a 2 g single dose.

Gardnerella vaginalis or bacterial vaginosis (previously known as Haemophilus vaginalis)

- Bacterial vaginosis is a change in vaginal flora. It is a vaginal infection caused by a mixed group of organisms including *G. vaginalis*, *Mycoplasma hominis* and anaerobic organisms.

Presentation

- In women, there is a smelly, greyish, irritant vaginal discharge.

- It may be itchy. There is a fishy-smelling odour.

Diagnosis

- The diagnosis of bacterial vaginosis is made when three out of four of the following are present:

  - a smelly, greyish, irritant vaginal discharge, which may be itchy

  - a fishy-smelling odour, particularly when potassium hydroxide is added

  - vaginal pH >4.7

  - clue cells (squamous epithelial cells plastered with bacteria).

Treatment

- Flagyl 400 mg bd patient and partner for 7 days, or a 2 g single dose.

- There may be an Antabuse-like effect with Flagyl.

- Recurrent infections are common and can be potentiated by soap and sperm, both of which are alkaline and inhibit vaginal lactobacilli. Condoms may be helpful.

Chlamydia

- This is the most common cause worldwide of non-gonococcal urethritis in men.

- In women, the cervix is infected. The infection may be eliminated, may be asymptomatic, or can spread to other genital organs to cause pelvic inflammatory disease. It is as common as gonococcus.

Presentation

- In men, there is mucopurulent urethral discharge and pain on urination, which may be severe. In some cases, there is a frequent need to pass urine, and also bladder pain.

- In women in whom the infection has spread, the patient is ill with fever, and has a painful and tender abdomen.

- In neonates there is red eye and mucopus in the presence of a 'cobblestone' appearance of the conjunctival epithelium.

Diagnosis

- Send endocervical and urethral swabs for culture in chlamydia (not viral) transport medium (available from the laboratory on request).

- Enzyme immunoassays are now superseded by the nucleic acid amplification test, which can be performed on a vaginal swab or first-catch morning urine sample (not MSU) and which is much more sensitive.

- The swab should be sent off immediately, but if this is not possible, it should be stored at 4°C.

- In men, discharge can be examined under the microscope; sediment from the urine sample can be examined microscopically after centrifugation; samples of discharge can be sent for culture.

- In neonates, pus should be removed and the underlying cells (e.g. conjunctival) sent for culture.

Treatment

- Oxytetracycline, doxycycline or minocycline plus metronidazole are used to treat women.

- Erythromycin, 500 mg qid for 7–14 days, is suitable for pregnant or lactating women.

Actinomyces-like organisms (ALOs)

- Reported in women who have had an intrauterine contraceptive device (IUCD) for many years. Rare in women with an IUCD for <1 year. Can occur several months after removal of an IUCD.

- ALO presence is related to duration of use of an IUCD. After 1 year, 1–2% of smears contain ALOs; after 3 years, 8–10%, and after 5 years, 20%.

- It can be asymptomatic.

Presentation

- It is most commonly asymptomatic.

- Symptoms consist of pain, dyspareunia and excessive discharge.

Treatment

- If *symptomatic*, the IUCD should be removed and sent to the laboratory with an endocervical swab for culture. If symptoms persist, refer the patient to a gynaecologist.

- If *asymptomatic*, continue with the IUCD and advise the patient to return if specific symptoms arise. Repeat the smear as per routine.

  - OR remove the IUCD and replace it with a copper one. Repeat the smear in 3–12 months.

  - OR leave the IUCD *in situ* and treat the patient with penicillin or doxycycline. Repeat the smear after the course of treatment has ended.

- Where ALOs continue to be reported in an asymptomatic patient, an alternative form of contraception should be sought where possible.

Syphilis

- This is caused by the spirochaete *Treponema pallidum*.

- This disease has three stages – primary, secondary and tertiary. The tertiary stage is now rarely seen.

- All suspected cases should be referred.

Presentation

- In primary syphilis, a hard-edged ulcer, known as a *chancre*, is seen on the man's penis or on the woman's vulva. Lymph nodes in the groin may be swollen.

- In secondary syphilis, the affected individual feels ill and may have headaches and joint pains. There is a pale skin rash that persists for 6 weeks and then fades slowly. A few subjects develop ulcers in the mouth, vulva or anus.

Diagnosis

- Refer the patient to a genito-urinary clinic if possible.

- A sample of clear fluid taken from the centre of a cleaned chancre is examined under the microscope to detect treponemas.

- Blood tests for syphilis are negative for about 6 weeks after infection.

- If the Venereal Disease Reference Laboratory (VDRL) or *Treponema pallidum* haemagglutination assay test is positive, the FTAABS (fluorescent treponemal antibody absorption test) is used to confirm the diagnosis.

- False-positive results on the VDRL test may occur:
  - after typhoid or yellow fever immunisation
  - following an acute febrile illness
  - in pregnancy
  - in autoimmune disease (rheumatoid arthritis and systemic lupus erythematosus)
  - in other treponemal infections (e.g. yaws)
  - in some malignancies.

- The VDRL test becomes negative after treatment.

- The *Treponema pallidum* haemagglutination assay test may be used for screening instead of the VDRL test.

- The FTAABS is highly specific and remains positive for years after infection.

Treatment
- Penicillin is used for treatment.

- Follow-up blood tests for 12 months after treatment are essential.

  NB: If neither primary nor secondary syphilis is treated, tertiary syphilis may develop 2–20 years after infection. This is a serious condition that carries a high risk of death at an early age, and is characterised by damage to many different tissues.

Group B streptococci
- These are occasionally seen on HVSs.

- They are the commonest cause of neonatal sepsis but treatment does not eradicate carriage and does not usually require treatment.

- Coliforms and anaerobic cocci are also normal vaginal flora.

- It is useful at delivery to know that a woman has been a carrier to determine the need for prophylaxis in labour.

UTI

- Clean-catch MSU samples should be obtained from all pregnant women, children and men with symptoms of dysuria and/or frequency.

- Otherwise, MSU samples need only be taken from patients who have complicated infections, or for whom standard treatment has failed.

- Proteinuria is a poor guide to infection. Although nitrite stick tests are better, they still have a poor sensitivity (i.e. too many false-negative results).

- Asymptomatic bacteriuria is common in the elderly, is not usually clinically significant and does not require or respond to treatment.

- The criteria for UTI are two of fever, frequency, dysuria or suprapubic pain on palpation *and* dipstix positive leucocyte esterase or nitrate. Where an MSU is taken, definite infection is confirmed by $>10^5$ organisms/ml, with >100 white cells per high-power field.

- If there are >100 white cells with *no* organisms, *consider*:

  - venereal disease

  - malignancy

  - tuberculosis (TB)

  - post-irradiation kidney stones.

  NB: Catheter infections rarely require treatment unless the patient is symptomatic, i.e. rigors, new onset of delirium, or temperature >38°C or 1.5°C above baseline on two occasions over 12 hours. Cultures will be positive in many catheter specimens unless patients were only recently catheterised (in the preceding 2–3 days).

FUNGAL NAIL DISEASE

- Fungal nail disease (onychomycosis) is a relatively common chronic fungal infection and a frequent cause of nail deformity. The vast majority of infections are caused by one of three species of dermatophyte fungi:

  - *Trichophyton rubrum*

- *T. interdigitale*

- *Epidermophyton floccosum.*

- Occasionally there are mixed infections and other dermatophyte fungi, e.g. *T. erinacei, T. tonsurans.*

- Candida species (yeasts) are a rare cause of nail infections but most are caused by *Candida albicans*. Even with a positive microscopy and pure growth on culture, it is still difficult to determine their significance.

- Non-dermatophyte moulds are frequently cultured from samples of dystrophic nails, but in the majority of cases they are there simply as saprophytic organisms. More often than not, the primary cause of such nail dystrophy is a dermatophyte infection that may be masked in culture by overgrowth of the mould. In these cases, treatment of the dermatophyte will allow normal nail growth and saprophytic moulds will simply disappear.

- *Scopulariopsis brevicaulis* is the commonest non-dermatophyte mould cultured from nails in the UK. The organism is unlikely to be a primary pathogen and most often coexists with a dermatophyte.

- *Scytalidium dimidiatum* (formerly *Hendersonula toruloidea*) is the only non-dermatophyte mould that is a primary pathogen of nails. The pattern of nail infection is the same as with other dermatophytes although *Scytalidium* produces characteristic black discolouration of the nail. The mould doesn't respond well to antifungal therapy and in some cases removal of the nail may be the only effective management.

- Other moulds may cause significant infection in some immunosuppressed patients and advice in this patient group should be sought from a consultant microbiologist.

OTHER ORGANISMS
Streptococcus

- *Streptococcus pyogenes* is the most common bacterial cause of pharyngitis.

- Antistreptolysin-O (ASO) has a normal range of <200 IU/ml.

Diagnosis

- The ASO titre can confirm infection with *Streptococcus* 2–6 weeks after the organism may have disappeared.

- An ASO titre should be requested in any condition in which *Streptococcus* is thought to be responsible for the illness (e.g. arthralgia with or without haematuria, glomerulonephritis, rheumatic fever, erythema nodosum, Stevens–Johnson syndrome).

- Titres of >200 indicate possible recent streptococcal illness.

- It is ideal to detect a rise in titres over two tests separated by an interval of 2 weeks.

- A rise in titres indicates recent streptococcal illness.

  NB: Several other Gram-positive organisms may cause a similar rise in titres.

Treatment

- Due to the risk of bacterial endocarditis and glomerulonephritis (Lancefield Group A), more severe cases are treated with penicillin, although milder and asymptomatic cases probably do not require treatment.

Toxoplasmosis

- The protozoal parasite responsible for infection is *Toxoplasma gondii*.

- In most cases, affected individuals are asymptomatic or have only subclinical or mild infection.

- Unsuspected infection in pregnancy can be passed from the mother to her unborn child in up to 50% of cases.

- This infection is of increasing importance in immunocompromised individuals.

Skin and wound organisms

- Swabs may be taken from skin or wounds if there is a suspicion of cellulitis or pus is present.

- The following organisms may be found:
  - Diphtheroids   normal skin flora
  - Bacteroides   most common gut flora, usually a contaminant

- Coliforms   gut flora which are uncommon in a wound
                   infection and only require treatment if there is
                   cellulitis or if the patient is diabetic.

Presentation

- In acute illness, there is pneumonia with fever, cough,
  generalised aches and pains, malaise, maculopapular rash
  and lymphadenopathy with lymphocytosis showing atypical
  mononuclear cells similar to those in glandular fever.

- Rarely there is jaundice and myocarditis.

- It can cause choroidoretinitis and uveitis in adults.

- Infection passed to the child *in utero* can cause encephalomyelitis,
  hydrocephalus, microcephaly, cerebral calcification and
  choroidoretinitis.

- It may present with prolonged malaise and has been associated
  with myalgic encephalomyelitis.

Diagnosis

- Antibodies detectable by fluorescence or dye test appear early in
  the disease and persist for years.

- Complement-fixing antibodies appear late and decline more quickly.

- Around 20–40% of normal adults give positive latex test at titres of
  1/8–1/128.

- A titre of 1/256 can be expected in 1% of adults.

- Any titre, however low, should be regarded as indicating infection
  at some time in the past.

- Negative results are uncommon, and are therefore useful in
  excluding the disease.

- Antibodies may not be detectable in ocular toxoplasmosis. In ocular
  toxoplasmosis, some cases may give titres of about 1/256, but the
  majority of them are in the range 1/8–1/128.

- In pregnancy, IgM determination can be useful for detecting recent
  infection.

Treatment
- Usually only treated in immunosuppressed individuals.
- Sulphonamide, 1 g qds, and pyrimethamine, 25 mg daily for 2 weeks, are used in all active cases.
- Supplements of folic acid are required.
- Tetracycline, 250 mg qds for 4 weeks, should be given if the sulphonamide and pyrimethamine combination ineffective treatment fails.
- For uveitis and choroidoretinitis, use corticosteroids.
- Clindamycin is a newer alternative.

Measles and rubella antibodies
- Saliva testing is sometimes performed to determine a recent infection with measles.
- IgM antibody indicates an acute recent infection and IgG indicates past infection or previous vaccination and therefore prior immunity.

Chicken pox in pregnancy
- If a woman develops chicken pox while she is pregnant (up to 20 weeks' gestation), the baby is at risk of developing foetal varicella syndrome.
- Maternal chicken pox between 1 week before and 1 week after delivery exposes the baby to neonatal varicella.
- The serum of a pregnant woman can be tested at any time for *Varicella zoster* virus antibody and, if it is absent, immunoglobulin may be recommended given if the patient is nonimmune.

CEREBROSPINAL FLUID (CSF)
- Normal range (mm^3): <5 lymphocyte cells.
  - Red or white blood cell counts ($\times 10^6$/l): <1
  - (g/l): 0.1–0.5 protein
  - (mmol/l): 2.1–4.5 glucose (or no higher than 60% of blood sugar)
  - Culture: no growth.

- The sample (5 ml) is divided into three tubes, one containing fluoride for glucose estimation.

Abnormal test results
- 10^3–10^4 mm polymorphs predominant, protein up to 3 and lowered blood sugar suggests bacterial infection.
- Up to 4,000 cells, lymphocytes predominant, protein raised to 1–6 and blood sugar 1–4 mmol/l suggests TB.
- 10–20,000 cells/mm^3, lymphocytes present, protein up to 1.5 and normal blood sugar suggests viral infection.
- Raised CSF glucose suggests post-infectious encephalitis, tumours, uraemia, diabetic coma.
- Lowered CSF glucose suggests bacterial meningitis, TB, syphilis, insulin therapy.

CSF pressure
- Normal range: 70–200 mm of water.

Abnormal test results
- Raised values:
  - viral meningitis or encephalitis
  - subdural haemorrhage
  - subarachnoid haemorrhage
  - alcoholism.
- Very high values suggest:
  - bacterial meningitis
  - syphilis
  - TB
  - cerebral haemorrhage
  - toxoplasmosis.

TABLE 2.1 Cerebrospinal fluid

	Pressure	Gross appearance	Cells (×10⁶/l)	Protein [g/l]	Protein [mg/100 ml]	Globulin test	Chlorides as sodium chloride [mmol/l]	Chlorides [mg/100 ml]	Glucose [mmol/l]	Glucose [mg/100 ml]	Lange curve	Wasserman reaction
Normal	70–200 mm water	Clear, colourless	0–8	0.1–0.45	10–45	Negative	120–128	700–750	2.5–4.7	45–85	–	–
Pyogenic meningitis	Increased	Turbid or purulent	1,000–2,000+	0.5–5.0	50–500	Positive	111–120	850–700	0–2.5	0–45	'Meningitic'	–
Tuberculous meningitis	Increased	Clear or cobweb clot	100–300 (mostly lymphocytes)	0.5–1.0	50–100	Usually positive	86–103	500–600	0.8–2.5	15–45	Sometimes 'meningitic'	–
Acute aseptic meningitis	Increased	Clear or cloudy	50–1,500 (lymphocytes)	Increased	Increased	Positive	Normal	Normal	Normal	Normal	–	–
Poliomyelitis	Increased	Clear	50–250 (polymorphs then lymphocytes)	0.5–2.0	50–200	Positive	Normal	Normal	Normal	Normal	–	–
Subarachnoid haemorrhage	Increased	Bloody, xanthochromic	Increased (lymphocytes)	0.5–1.0	50–100	–	–	–	–	–	–	–

CSF colour

- Yellow suggests:
  - old haemorrhage and/or
  - high protein content.
- Red suggests:
  - recent haemorrhage
  - traumatic tap.
- Cloudy suggests:
  - high cell count.

Chapter 3

Fertility and pregnancy testing

FEMALE HORMONE PROFILES

- Measurement of female hormone levels (usually on day 22 of the menstrual cycle) can indicate whether ovulation has occurred.

- Follicle-stimulating hormone (FSH), luteinising hormone (LH), prolactin, testosterone and thyroid function should be measured between days 2 and 6 in the investigation of infertility in women with irregular menstrual cycles, i.e. <24 or >35 days.

Serum LH

- Normal range in women (µmol/l):

  - follicular phase, 0.8–9.0

  - mid-cycle, ≤65

  - luteal phase, 0.7–14.5.

- LH in men, 1.7–8.6 IU/l.

- In men with low testosterone, LH will determine whether hypogonadism is present or not and whether it is primary or secondary.

Abnormal test results

- In women LH is raised in:

    - polycystic ovarian syndrome (PCOS), as is serum testosterone, and LH/FSH ratio is increased.

- Sex-hormone-bonding globulins (SHBGs) are decreased in PCOS.

- Levels are *low* in:

    - pituitary failure

    - anorexia nervosa.

Serum follicle-stimulating hormone (FSH)

- Normal range (IU/l):

    - follicular phase, 2.5–9.7

    - mid-cycle, up to 7.6–19

    - luteal phase, 0.9–5.8

    - post-menopause, 12–100.

Abnormal test results

- FSH levels are *raised* in:

    - ovarian dysfunction (e.g. premature menopause, 15–30).

- FSH levels are *lowered* in:

    - pituitary failure

    - pituitary adenomas

    - PCOS.

Serum testosterone

- Normal range in women (nmol/l):

    - 0.3–2.8 (pre-menopause)

    - 0.3–1.2 (post-menopause).

- Normal range in men: 8.3–27.8 nmol/l.

- Testosterone should be measured on early morning (before 1100 hours) sample.

- Testosterone levels decline with age.

- In men, if testosterone is >12 but <28 nmol/l, no action is required.

- If testosterone >28 or <7 nmol/l, refer for investigation.

- If testosterone 7–12, repeat test.

- Obesity is the commonest cause of declining testosterone and weight loss can increase testosterone.

- Co-morbidities such as type 2 diabetes and COPD may cause low testosterone.

- If referring to hospital, check SHBG, thyroid-stimulating hormone (TSH), LH, FSH and prolactin.

Abnormal test result

- An LH/FSH ratio of >3:1 suggests polycystic disease.

- Raised testosterone in a female (>6 nmol/l) suggests a neoplastic cause. REFER female patients with serum testosterone >5 nmol/l for further investigation.

- Other causes include:

  - PCOS

  - Cushing's syndrome

  - hypothyroidism

  - adrenogenital syndrome

  - drug-induced causes (e.g. phenytoin, progesterone, diazoxide).

- When measuring plasma testosterone, the serum SHBG may also be measured (normal range in men is 10–50 nmol/l). As the level of SHBG increases, so usually does the testosterone level. If the plasma testosterone level is raised and the SHBG level remains normal, or at the lower end of the normal range, then a true excess of androgen exists, as in PCOS (which may be confirmed by ultrasound examination of the ovaries).

Free androgen index (FAI)

- $\text{FAI} = \dfrac{plasma\ testosterone}{\text{SHBG}} \times 100$

- Normal range = 1–10.

- SHBG and FAI are similar to thyroxine-binding globulin (TBG) and free thyroxine index in thyroid function tests (TFT) (*see* p. 149).

- SHBG varies with the menstrual cycle, and is raised in:
  - women taking the oral contraceptive pill
  - pregnancy
  - hyperthyroidism.

Plasma progesterone

- Measure plasma progesterone 7 days before onset of *next* period.
- Normal range (nmol/l):
  - >30 indicates normal ovulation
  - <16 indicates *no* ovulation
  - 16–30 repeat test
  - post-menopause, 0.1–1.0.

Plasma oestradiol

- Normal range (pmol/l):
  - follicular phase, 40–170
  - mid-cycle, 440–1,400
  - luteal phase, 180–1,000
  - post-menopause, 35–175.

Investigations of female fertility

- LH/FSH within the first 5 days of menses
  - high LH or high LH/FSH ratio suggestive of polycystic ovaries
  - high FSH suggestive of ovarian resistance or failure
  - low FSH or LH suggestive of hypothalamic dysfunction.

- Progesterone
    - day 21 of a 28-day cycle (7 days before expected ovulation) low progesterone may imply problem with ovulation, repeat test.
- TSH
    - thyroid disease can impair fertility.
- Testosterone
    - high level may suggest polycystic ovaries.
- SHBG
    - low levels may indicate polycystic ovaries.
- Prolactin
    - high levels may indicate pituitary tumour.

Menopause

- Serum FSH and LH levels are both raised, while the plasma oestradiol level is lowered, i.e. oestradiol is in the range 100–200 pmol/l and FSH is >15–20 (often >30) IU/l.
- FSH >30 indicates permanent ovarian failure, e.g. post-menopause.
- 15–30 indicates peri-menopause.

Serum prolactin

- Normal range (mU/l):
    - male, <20 mU/l
    - female in follicular phase, <23 or up to 610 mU/l.
- Conditions that cause raised levels of prolactin include:
    - physiological causes
    - pregnancy and lactation
    - craniopharyngioma
    - hypothyroidism
    - renal failure
    - stress
    - PCOS.

- Drugs that cause raised levels of prolactin include cimetidine, haloperidol, methyldopa, metoclopramide, oestrogens, phenothiazines, domperidone, antihistamines and cannabis.

Abnormal test results
- Raised serum prolactin levels (>2,000 mU/l) strongly suggest pituitary adenoma.

- Raised prolactin levels (<2,000 mU/l) may be a finding in the following:

  - gynaecomastia

  - galactorrhoea

  - infertility

  - secondary amenorrhoea

  - impotence

  - dysfunctional bleeding, irregular cycle or amenorrhoea.

- REFER if levels >1,000.

Hirsutism
- PCOS, Cushing's syndrome, adrenal tumours and ovarian tumours may cause hirsutism (unwanted and excessive hair growth).

- Drugs such as ciclosporin, phenytoin, danazol and diazoxide may cause hypertrichosis, as may hypothyroidism and anorexia nervosa.

Investigations in hirsutism
- Pregnancy test.

- FSH, LH, prolactin, testosterone, TFT.

- Testosterone >5 suggests androgen tumour.

- Testosterone >2.5 but <5 suggests PCOS.

- Pelvic USS to exclude pregnancy.

SEMEN ANALYSIS

- The initial investigation of male/female infertility involves assessment of the following:
  - total sperm count
  - sperm motility
  - volume of semen.
- Two *fresh* specimens, produced at least 7 days but less than 3 months apart, should be provided in a clean glass or plastic container (not in a condom) and taken to the laboratory for analysis within 1 hour.
- Each specimen should be obtained after abstaining from intercourse for a minimum of 2 days and a maximum of 7 days.
- Normal range:
  - sperm concentration >15 million/ml
  - total sperm numbers >39 million/ml
  - normal morphology >4%
  - total motility, 40% or above
  - progressive motility, 32% or above
  - volume, 1.5 ml
  - white blood cell count, <1 million/ml.
- Sperm motility is graded, 1 being least mobile and 3 being optimum (random) motility.
- Sperm morphology is of limited value in the assessment of infertility, but where figures are quoted they should show normal morphology and viability in over 50%.
- Factors that affect the sperm count:
  - warm testicles (suggest loose-fitting pants, avoiding hot baths, and weight loss where appropriate)
  - smoking
  - alcohol

- drugs (e.g. cimetidine, propranolol, spironolactone, sulphasalazine, anabolic steroids)

- varicocele (possibly).

Antisperm antibodies

- Circulating antisperm antibodies (IgG or IgM) may be sought or some specialised laboratories may detect antibodies in the seminal fluid or cervical mucus (IgA, IgG or IgM).

- Antisperm antibodies in one or both partners may account for up to 20% of cases of otherwise unexplained infertility.

- Antisperm antibodies are of doubtful significance when found in the serum alone. When present in the seminal plasma, titres of ≤1:32 are unlikely to have an adverse effect on fertility, but higher levels are likely to have such an effect.

- High antisperm antibodies: REFER for in vitro fertilisation.

Erectile dysfunction

- Organic causes of impotence may be neurological (e.g. multiple sclerosis), vascular (e.g. arteriosclerosis) or endocrine.

- The key endocrine disorders which should be considered in the investigation of impotence are:

  - diabetes (*see* p. 142), 50% of men with diabetes are impotent

  - hyperprolactinaemia (*see* p. 77)

  - thyroid disorders (*see* p. 149).

- A low serum testosterone level can lead to impotence, but the effect on erectile function of declining testosterone with age is uncertain.

- The following drugs may cause erectile dysfunction:

  - antihypertensives (e.g. thiazide diuretics, beta-blockers and angiotensin-converting enzyme inhibitors)

  - antidepressants (e.g. tricyclic antidepressants and monoamine oxidase inhibitors)

  - major tranquillisers (e.g. phenothiazines)

  - anti-androgens (e.g. finasteride, cyproterone acetate, flutamide)

- psychotropic drugs (e.g. alcohol, barbiturates, amphetamines and marijuana).

PREGNANCY TESTS

- Urine pregnancy tests measure beta-human chorionic gonadotrophin (HCG).

  NB: Urinary HCG pregnancy tests do not work after 20 weeks' gestation, and should not be relied on to exclude pregnancy after a few months of amenorrhoea.

- The first morning specimen should be tested; if an unexpected negative result is obtained, a random sample should be tested and checked against the early-morning sample.

- Specimens may be stored in a refrigerator and tested within 72 hours.

- Less than 50% of tests are positive in extrauterine (i.e. ectopic) pregnancies.

- In cases where an ectopic pregnancy is suspected, the serum HCG should be requested, which is 200 times more sensitive.

- A persistently raised serum HCG of >1,000, on consecutive days, in the absence of an intrauterine pregnancy on ultrasound test is highly suggestive of an ectopic pregnancy.

- Serum HCG is checked after exactly 48 hours, and if it has risen but not doubled, this is also suggestive of an ectopic pregnancy. A rapidly falling serum HCG is strongly suggestive of a miscarriage.

- A urinary pregnancy test will detect >50 IU of beta-HCG and a serum test will detect >5 IU. Serum beta-HCG and pelvic ultrasound have a positive predictive value of over 90%.

- Serum HCG of <2 indicates that pregnancy is unlikely.

- Patients who have repeated false-positive tests should have their serum HCG levels measured in order to check for chorion carcinoma.

RHESUS BLOOD GROUP TESTING

- All rhesus-negative mothers with transfusions and/or an obstetric history associated with haemolytic disease of the newborn (HDN), such as three consecutive miscarriages at less than 20 weeks, one miscarriage/termination of pregnancy at more than 20 weeks, or a stillborn infant, jaundiced infant or unexplained neonatal death, should be tested.

- Samples are required before the 12th week, at the 28th and 36th week, and at delivery.

- Rhesus-positive women with a transfusion history also require regular samples (5 ml clotted and 5 ml anticoagulated samples are required in each case).

Scheme for sampling pre- and postnatally

- This should be performed for all known rhesus-negative women and rhesus-positive women who have a history of transfusion and/ or an obstetric history associated with HDN since they were last tested.

- Sample required 6 months postnatally:
  - rhesus-negative women delivered of a rhesus-positive infant.

- Sample required at next pregnancy:
  - rhesus-negative women delivered of a rhesus-negative infant.

- No further samples required:
  - rhesus-positive women with no transfusion or obstetric history.

Kleihauer test

- All rhesus-negative women should be tested within 24 hours of a threatened miscarriage, miscarriage, termination of pregnancy, or after abdominal trauma that may result in the transplacental transfer of blood cells.

- Foetal cells are looked for and a dose of anti-D administered (250 or 500 IU within 72 hours).

- Some centres now give anti-D at 28 and 36 weeks in the antenatal period, even in cases where there has been no risk of transplacental transfer of cells.

ALPHA-FETOPROTEINS (AFPs)

- AFP may be measured in serum or in amniotic fluid.

- During pregnancy, measurement of serum AFP is a routine screening test performed in most (but not all) centres.

- Used to detect neural-tube defects and Down's syndrome, it may also be of value in predicting twin pregnancies and intrauterine growth retardation.

- In non-pregnant patients, serum AFP may also be used to monitor liver disease and gonadal cancer.

- Seminoma is AFP negative.

- 90% of teratomas have an elevated AFP or beta-HCG.

Normal serum values in pregnancy (µg/l)

- 16 weeks' gestation:

  - 26.5 mean

  - <10–53, range

  - >64, neural-tube defect is likely.

- 17 weeks' gestation:

  - 31 mean

  - <10–62, range

  - >74, neural-tube defect is likely.

- 18 weeks' gestation:

  - 34.5 mean

  - <10–69, range

  - >83, neural-tube defect is likely.

Abnormal test results

- Raised serum AFP suggests open neural-tube defects or trisomy 21.

  NB: A detailed ultrasound scan of the foetus is the usual secondary investigation.

- Lowered serum AFP may suggest Down's syndrome.

- The level of AFP in the amniotic fluid falls steadily throughout pregnancy.

Normal range for amniotic AFP (kU/l)

- 16 weeks' gestation, 8–24.

- 18 weeks' gestation, 7–23.

- 20 weeks' gestation, 3–16.

Abnormal test results

- Raised amniotic AFP may indicate the following:

  - foetal distress

  - neural-tube defect

  - twins.

- Lowered amniotic AFP is found in Down's syndrome.

The triple test

- The serum AFP level, together with levels of unconjugated oestriol and HCG, is expressed as a multiple of the median level for a normal pregnancy of the same gestation. A computer-assisted interpretation of the result also takes into account the mother's age.

- Information required by the laboratory includes:

  - gestational age, preferably based on a scan

  - maternal weight

  - previous history of neural-tube defect or Down's syndrome

  - history of twin pregnancy or insulin-dependent diabetes in current pregnancy.

- The triple test is positive in 1 in 250 tests. This represents a 58% detection rate (for Down's syndrome) overall, or an 89% rate for mothers over the age of 37 years.

- The test is of limited value because of its low specificity and sensitivity.

Serum AFP in non-pregnant adults

Abnormal test results

- AFP levels of >500 µg/l suggest primary hepatoma.

- AFP levels of <500 µg/l suggest:

  - primary or secondary hepatoma

  - cirrhosis

  - hepatitis

  - cancer of the gastrointestinal tract

  - cancer of the ovaries or testicles.

Plasma oestriols (during pregnancy)

- Normal range (nmol/l):

  - 32 weeks, 145–800

  - 34 weeks, 170–1040

  - 36 weeks, 230–1400

  - 38 weeks, 300–1560

  - 40 weeks, 350–1600.

- Single tests are of little value, but a trend such as falling levels is indicative of foetal distress. Levels should rise during pregnancy, and therefore the absence of such an increase should indicate the possibility of foetal distress.

- Steroids and ampicillin can depress plasma oestriol values.

Chapter 4

Rheumatology and immunology

TESTING FOR RHEUMATOID ARTHRITIS (RA)

The following tests may be of diagnostic help in distinguishing the many forms of RA.

Erythrocyte sedimentation rate (ESR)
See p. 17.

Plasma viscosity
See p. 16.

C-reactive protein
See p. 18.

RA latex test

- May use latex beads coated with altered human immunoglobulin or sheep red cells coated with rabbit immunoglobulin. Either test positive titre of 1:32 or more (titre of 1:64 is significant, whereas titre of 1:16 is not significant).

- The test is negative in 20–25% of patients, especially in the early stages of the disease.

Rose–Waaler test

- The rheumatoid arthritis haemagglutination assay (RAHA) test has replaced the Rose–Waaler test for RA in many laboratories.

Rheumatoid factors

- Rheumatoid factor is an IgM immunoglobulin.

- Patients with early RA often have a negative rheumatoid factor.

- The diagnosis of RA should be made on clinical grounds, not just on the basis of a blood test.

- About 80% of patients with RA will develop a positive test for IgM rheumatoid factor.

- About 10% of the elderly population have a positive titre with no evidence of inflammatory joint disease.

- A RAHA titre of 1:80 is equivalent to a Rose–Waaler (SCAT/ DAT) titre of 1:16.

- The RAHA test is positive in 80% of rheumatoid patients.

- There is a false-positive rate of 5% in the normal population.

Test results
- A titre of 1:80 is weakly positive.

- A titre of 1:160 is significant.

- Rheumatoid factor (IU/ml):

  - <15   negative

  - 15–30   borderline

  - 30–100   weak positive

  - 100–400   positive

  - >400   strong positive.

Differential diagnosis
- If a patient with suspected RA is sero-negative (i.e. negative RAHA), obtain further information from X-rays, where RA may be distinguished from psoriasis and osteoarthritis once disease has been present for 1–2 years.

- Rheumatoid factors (usually at lower levels) can be found less frequently in other connective tissue diseases (CTDs) (e.g. lupus, primary biliary cirrhosis, Sjögren's syndrome, chronic infective endocarditis and tuberculosis).

Antinuclear antibodies (ANAs)

- These are indicated in the investigation of suspected CTD.

- Normal range (IU/ml) is 0–25 (titre 0:10).

- ANAs are probably best reserved for young women with features suggestive of systemic lupus erythematosus (SLE) or other CTDs, e.g. scleroderma.

- ANA is often present in older patients and is present in 80–90% of patients with SLE, so is the best screening test for SLE.

- ANA is positive in 70–80% of patients with scleroderma.

- 5% of normal population are positive for ANA.

Test results

- In RA, the presence of ANAs may suggest:

  - Felty's syndrome

  - Sjögren's syndrome.

- ANAs are present in 20–40% of patients with RA, but are more a pointer to other CTDs such as:

  - SLE

  - juvenile chronic arthritis

  - Sjögren's syndrome

  - fibrosing alveolitis

  - viral infections (Epstein–Barr virus (EBV), cytomegalovirus)

  - uveitis

  - chronic liver disease

  - pneumoconioses

  - drug reactions

  - relatives of patients with SLE.

DNA antibody

- This is mainly positive in patients with SLE and may correlate with disease activity.

Complement

- Single-point measurements of complement are of limited value; serial levels are much more useful.

- Normal range (g/l):

  - plasma C_3, 0.63–1.70

  - plasma C_4, 0.11–0.45.

- Anti-dsDNA antibody:

  - <20 IU/ml　negative

  - >20 IU/ml　positive.

Test results

- Raised C_3 and normal C_4 indicates an acute-phase response (e.g. RA).

- Low C_3 and/or C_4 suggests immune-complex-mediated disease (e.g. glomerulonephritis due to immune-complex disease) or complement activation, and may be found in:

  - SLE (during relapse).

- Decreased C_3 in the presence of normal C_4 is seen in Gram-negative septicaemia and membranoproliferative glomerulonephritis.

- Normal or raised C_4 occurs in RA.

- In hereditary angioedema, C_4 levels are decreased during attacks while C_3 levels remain normal.

C_{3d}

This degradation product of C_3 is elevated in conditions that cause complement activation, such as SLE.

C_1 esterase inhibitor (C_{1EI})

Low levels (30–50% of normal) are found in 85% of patients with congenital hereditary angioedema.

C-reactive protein (CRP)

CRP is an acute-phase protein, which is elevated in acute inflammatory conditions, including bacterial infections, tissue damage and inflammation.

CRP can be useful in differentiating between connective tissue disorders (CTD) and monitoring RA activity.

- It is a non-specific test indicating:

  - tissue inflammation

  - damage

  - necrosis

  - organic disease.

- It is more sensitive than ESR.

- It is useful for monitoring the activity of RA.

- Normal range, 0–5:

  - mild inflammation/viral infection, up to 40

  - active inflammation/bacterial infection, 40–200

  - serious bacterial infection, up to 500.

- CRP may be raised in RA when ESR remains normal.

- CRP may be normal in SLE when ESR is raised.

Human leucocyte antigen (HLA) B27

Test results

- This is a positive test in:

  - ankylosing spondylitis

  - Reiter's disease

  - juvenile chronic polyarthritis

  - post-infection arthritis

  - inflammatory bowel disease

  - acute anterior uveitis.

- Because it is positive in 8% of the normal population who do not have ankylosing spondylitis, the HLA test is not a good screening test for ankylosing spondylitis but can be used to confirm the diagnosis when the history, examination and X-ray findings are equivocal.

HEPATITIS B

- The diagnosis of acute hepatitis is made by detecting HbsAg and IgM antibody to hepatitis B core antigen (anti-HbcAg) in a patient with other biochemical evidence of acute hepatitis.

  - HBsAg   indicates current infection

  - HBeAg   indicates active viral replication

  - Anti-HBsAg   indicates immunity following infection or post-immunisation

  - Anti-HBcAg IgM   indicates acute current infection

  - Anti-HBcAg IgG   indicates past infection or chronic ongoing infection.

AUTOANTIBODIES

The autoantibody screen usually includes antinuclear, antithyroid, antimitochondrial, antigastric parietal cell and anti-smooth muscle autoantibodies.

CREST is a localised form of systemic sclerosis comprising:

- **C**alcinosis – palpable nodules in the hands due to calcium deposits in the subcutaneous tissue

- **R**aynaud's phenomenon

- **O**esophageal dysmotility

- **S**clerodactyly – tightening of the skin of the fingers

- **T**elangiectasia – often multiple, large and on the fingers.

CREST may be suggested by an autoimmune screen which demonstrates ANA **centromere specificity**.

Antinuclear antibodies
See p. 89.

Antithyroid antibodies
Elevated titres of antithyroid microsomal antibodies with or without elevated titres of antithyroglobulin antibodies are found in primary myxoedema, Hashimoto's thyroiditis and Graves' disease. Elevated titres may precede overt clinical thyroid disease, and serial thyroid function tests should be performed.

Antimitochondrial antibodies
High titres occur in 95% of patients with primary biliary cirrhosis, but low titres may also be found in patients with chronic active hepatitis.

Antigastric parietal antibodies
Gastric parietal antibodies are present in 95% of patients with pernicious anaemia, but are also present in 3% of the normal population, and the incidence rises with increasing age. Anti-intrinsic factor antibodies are also likely to be raised.

Anti-intrinsic factor antibodies
Anti-intrinsic factor antibodies are present in 75% of patients with pernicious anaemia.

Anti-smooth muscle antibodies
• High titres are associated with autoimmune chronic active hepatitis (therefore check liver function tests (LFT), including albumin and international normalised ratio).

• Low titres may occur in viral infections, especially EBV and hepatitis A, and usually disappear within a few months.

Antigliadin antibodies
This is a screening test for coeliac disease and dermatitis herpetiformis. Where positive results are obtained, anti-endomysial antibodies may also be assayed.

Anti-endomysial antibodies
These confirm the presence of coeliac disease and/or dermatitis herpetiformis.
Testing for anti-endomysial antibody is the screening test of choice,

though it can be negative in up to 20% of patients with coeliac disease. If the diagnosis is strongly suspected, consider requesting total IgA quantification and IgG class antibody test. Despite a negative endomysial antibody, referral for consideration of small bowel biopsy should be considered.

Serological screening tests revert back to normal when the patient is on a gluten-free diet.

Anti-glomerular basement membrane antibodies
This test is positive in 90% of patients with Goodpasture's syndrome.

Anti-islet-cell antibodies
This test is predictive of future insulin requirement in patients with non-insulin-dependent diabetes mellitus and in the relatives of patients with insulin-dependent diabetes mellitus.

Anti-acetylcholine-receptor antibodies
This test is positive in 80–90% of patients with myasthenia gravis.

Anti-skeletal muscle antibodies
These are associated with thymomatous myasthenia gravis, but they also occur in hepatitis viral infections and polymyositis.

Anti-adrenal antibodies
These are present in 60–70% of patients with idiopathic Addison's disease, and in cases of autoimmune premature ovarian failure.

Anti-cardiac muscle antibodies
These occur in some patients with Dressler's syndrome and post-cardiomyotomy syndrome.

Anti-centromere antibody
This is used in the investigation of Raynaud's phenomenon. The test is positive in 60–70% of cases of the CREST (*see* p. 92) variant of scleroderma and in 20% of cases of generalised scleroderma.

Antineutrophil cytoplasmic antibodies (ANCAs)
These are indicated in the investigation of vasculitis. Two patterns exist (cANCA and pANCA). cANCA is present in 90% of patients with Wegener's granuloma. pANCA is less specific but is associated with microscopic polyarteritis.

Antiphospholipid antibodies

These are found in antiphospholipid syndrome, which is characterised by recurrent spontaneous abortion, recurrent thrombosis (arterial or venous) and thrombocytopenia. This may occur either as a syndrome or secondary to SLE (*see also* p. 89).

Anti-peripheral nerve antibodies

These are found in Guillain–Barré syndrome.

Acid glycoprotein

- Normal range 600–1200 mg/l.

- Acid glycoprotein is an acute-phase protein used as a marker of inflammatory bowel disease.

INITIATION AND MONITORING OF DISEASE-MODIFYING ANTI-RHEUMATIC DRUGS (DMARDs)

- Monitoring of DMARDs in the management of rheumatoid and psoriatic arthritis, psoriasis, connective tissue diseases and inflammatory bowel disease is now often shared between primary and secondary care under Local Enhanced Services. As well as regular monitoring of disease activity by measuring the ESR or CRP, a full blood count (FBC) should always be performed and treatment withheld if the patient complains of a sore throat.

- A high platelet count ($>400 \times 10^9$/l) is sometimes a sign of active RA and falls with treatment.

The following routine monitoring for individual drugs should be performed.

Leflunomide

Time taken to respond: 8–12 weeks.

Monitoring

- FBC (including Hb white cell count (WCC) and platelets before commencement of treatment), every 2 weeks for 6 months and then every 8 weeks.

- LFT every 4 weeks for 6 months and then every 8 weeks.

Stop treatment or consult rheumatologist

- total WCC <3.5 × 10^9/l

- or neutrophil count <2 × 10^9/l

- or platelets <140 × 10^9/l

- if alanine aminotransferase (ALT) rises more than 3 times normal, recheck after 72 hours and STOP treatment if still 3 times normal upper limit

- if ALT 2–3 times upper limit of normal, recheck after 72 hours and if still 2–3 times upper limit reduce dosage and recheck ALT every 2 weeks

- if ALT less than twice the upper limit of normal, recheck every 2 weeks and expect to normalise in time.

Sulphasalazine

- FBC (including Hb, WCC and platelets) before commencement of treatment and 4-weekly for the first 3 months then 3-monthly.

- Creatinine (or estimated glomerular filtration rate (eGFR)) alkaline phosphatase and ALT should be monitored every 4 weeks for the first 3 months then 3-monthly thereafter.

- Time taken to respond to drug: 3 months.

Stop treatment or consult rheumatologist

- total WCC <3.5 × 10^9/l

- or neutrophil count <2 × 10^9/l

- or platelets <140 × 10^9/l

- Mean corpuscular volume (MCV) >105 (check B_{12}, folate and thyroid-stimulating hormone (TSH) as well as discuss with rheumatologist)

- if serum creatinine increases to more than 30% of baseline measurement or eGFR <45, reduce or stop treatment and discuss with rheumatologist

- if ALT rises more than 3 times normal, recheck after 72 hours and STOP treatment if still 3 times normal upper limit

- if ALT 2–3 times upper limit of normal, recheck after 72 hours and if still 2–3 times upper limit reduce dosage and recheck ALT every 2 weeks

- if ALT less than twice the upper limit of normal, recheck every 2 weeks and expect to normalise in time.

Methotrexate

Every 2 weeks for 8 weeks then 1- to 2-monthly.

- FBC (including Hb, WCC, MCV and platelets) should be performed at week 1, week 3 and then monthly after initiation of treatment and after any increase in dose.

- Creatinine (or eGFR) alkaline phosphatase and ALT should also be monitored at week 1, week 3 and then monthly after initiation of treatment and after any increase in dose.

- Time taken to respond: 6–12 weeks.

Stop treatment or consult rheumatologist

- total WCC $<3.5 \times 10^9/l$

- or neutrophil count $<2 \times 10^9/l$

- or platelets $<140 \times 10^9/l$

- MCV >105 (check B_{12} folate and TSH as well as discuss with rheumatologist)

- if serum creatinine increases to more than 30% of baseline measurement or eGFR <45, reduce or stop treatment and discuss with rheumatologist

- serum albumin decrease

- if ALT rises more than 3 times normal, recheck after 72 hours and STOP treatment if still 3 times normal upper limit

- if ALT 2–3 times upper limit of normal, recheck after 72 hours and if still 2–3 times upper limit reduce dosage and recheck ALT every 2 weeks

- if ALT less than twice the upper limit of normal, recheck every 2 weeks and expect to normalise in time.

Ciclosporin

- FBC (including Hb, WCC, MCV and platelets) should be performed at week 1, week 3 and then monthly after initiation of treatment and after any increase in dose.

- Creatinine (or eGFR) alkaline phosphatase and ALT should also be monitored at week 1, week 3 and then monthly after initiation of treatment and after any increase in dose.

- Fasting blood cholesterol should also be measured (can increase with treatment).

- Time taken to respond: 12 weeks.

Stop treatment or consult rheumatologist

- total WCC $<3.5 \times 10^9/l$

- or neutrophil count $<2 \times 10^9/l$

- or platelets $<140 \times 10^9/l$

- if serum creatinine increases to more than 30% of baseline measurement or eGFR <45, reduce or stop treatment and discuss with rheumatologist

- rise in fasting cholesterol

- if ALT rises more than 3 times normal, recheck after 72 hours and STOP treatment if still 3 times normal upper limit

- if ALT 2–3 times upper limit of normal, recheck after 72 hours and if still 2–3 times upper limit, reduce dosage and recheck ALT every 2 weeks

- if ALT less than twice the upper limit of normal, recheck every 2 weeks and expect to normalise in time

- if ALT rises more than 2.5 times normal

- or total WCC $<3.5 \times 10^9/l$

- or neutrophil count $<2 \times 10^9/l$

- or platelets $<140 \times 10^9/l$

- or urinary proteinuria (greater than a trace)

- or microscopic haematuria is present

- if serum creatinine increases to more than 30% of baseline measurement, reduce or stop treatment and discuss with rheumatologist.

Gold

- FBC (including Hb, WCC, MCV and platelets) should be performed at week 1, week 3 and then monthly after initiation of treatment and after any increase in dose.

- Creatinine (or eGFR) alkaline phosphatase and ALT should also be monitored at week 1, week 3 and then monthly after initiation of treatment and after any increase in dose.

- Gold may cause eosinophilia (>0.04–0.44) (1–4%). Stop gold therapy for 1–2 weeks and then resume it at a lower dose.

Stop treatment or consult rheumatologist

- total WCC <3.5 × 10^9/l

- or neutrophil count <2 × 10^9/l

- or platelets <140 × 10^9/l

- MCV >105 (check B$_{12}$, folate and TSH as well as discuss with rheumatologist)

- if serum creatinine increases to more than 30% of baseline measurement or eGFR <45, reduce or stop treatment and discuss with rheumatologist

- if ALT rises more than 3 times normal, recheck after 72 hours and STOP treatment if still 3 times normal upper limit

- if ALT 2–3 times upper limit of normal, recheck after 72 hours and if still 2–3 times upper limit, reduce dosage and recheck ALT every 2 weeks

- if ALT less than twice the upper limit of normal, recheck every 2 weeks and expect to normalise in time.

Penicillamine

- FBC (including Hb, WCC, MCV and platelets) should be performed at week 1, week 3 and then monthly after initiation of treatment and after any increase in dose.

- Creatinine (or eGFR) and urinalysis for protein and blood.

- Penicillamine may cause eosinophilia (>0.04–0.44) (1–4%). Stop therapy for 1–2 weeks and then resume it at a lower dose.

Stop treatment or consult rheumatologist
- total WCC <3.5 × 10^9/l

- or neutrophil count <2 × 10^9/l

- or platelets <140 × 10^9/l

- 2 plusses of proteinuria

- if serum creatinine increases to more than 30% of baseline measurement or eGFR <45, reduce or stop treatment and discuss with rheumatologist.

Azathioprine
- FBC (including Hb, WCC, MCV and platelets) should be performed at week 1, week 3 and then monthly after initiation of treatment and after any increase in dose.

- Creatinine (or eGFR) alkaline phosphatase and ALT should also be monitored at week 1, week 3 and then monthly after initiation of treatment and after any increase in dose.

Stop treatment or consult rheumatologist
- total WCC <3.5 × 10^9/l

- or neutrophil count <2 × 10^9/l

- or platelets <140 × 10^9/l

- MCV >105 (check B_{12}, folate and TSH as well as discuss with rheumatologist)

- if serum creatinine increases to more than 30% of baseline measurement or eGFR <45, reduce or stop treatment and discuss with rheumatologist

- if ALT rises more than 3 times normal, recheck after 72 hours and STOP treatment if still 3 times normal upper limit

- if ALT 2–3 times upper limit of normal, recheck after 72 hours and if still 2–3 times upper limit, reduce dosage and recheck ALT every 2 weeks

- if ALT less than twice the upper limit of normal, recheck every 2 weeks and expect to normalise in time.

Hydroxychloroquine

- FBC (including Hb, WCC, MCV and platelets) should be performed at week 1, week 3 and then monthly after initiation of treatment and after any increase in dose.

- Creatinine (or eGFR) alkaline phosphatase and ALT should also be monitored at week 1, week 3 and then monthly after initiation of treatment and after any increase in dose.

Stop treatment or consult rheumatologist

- total WCC $<3.5 \times 10^9/l$

- or neutrophil count $<2 \times 10^9/l$

- or platelets $<140 \times 10^9/l$

- if serum creatinine increases to more than 30% of baseline measurement or eGFR <45, reduce or stop treatment and discuss with rheumatologist

- if ALT rises more than 3 times normal, recheck after 72 hours and STOP treatment if still 3 times normal upper limit

- if ALT 2–3 times upper limit of normal, recheck after 72 hours and if still 2–3 times upper limit, reduce dosage and recheck ALT every 2 weeks

- if ALT less than twice the upper limit of normal, recheck every 2 weeks and expect to normalise in time.

In addition, full ophthalmological testing should be done every 3 months on patients taking hydroxychloroquine.

Auranofin

- FBC (including Hb, WCC, MCV and platelets) should be performed at week 1, week 3 and then monthly after initiation of treatment and after any increase in dose.

- Check urine for protein and blood on each occasion. Creatinine (or eGFR) alkaline phosphatase and ALT should also be monitored at week 1, week 3 and then monthly after initiation of treatment and after any increase in dose.

- Auranofin may cause eosinophilia (>0.04–0.44) (1–4%). Stop therapy for 1–2 weeks and then resume it at a lower dose.

Stop treatment or consult rheumatologist
- total WCC <3.5 × 10⁹/l
- or neutrophil count <2 × 10⁹/l
- or platelets <140 × 10⁹/l
- if serum creatinine increases to more than 30% of baseline measurement or eGFR <45, reduce or stop treatment and discuss with rheumatologist
- 2 plusses of proteinuria
- if ALT rises more than 3 times normal, recheck after 72 hours and STOP treatment if still 3 times normal upper limit
- if ALT 2–3 times upper limit of normal, recheck after 72 hours and if still 2–3 times upper limit, reduce dosage and recheck ALT every 2 weeks
- if ALT less than twice the upper limit of normal, recheck every 2 weeks and expect to normalise in time.

Sodium aurothiomalate
- FBC (including Hb, WCC, MCV and platelets) should be performed at week 1, week 3 and then monthly after initiation of treatment and after any increase in dose.

- Check urine for protein and blood each time.

- Creatinine (or eGFR) alkaline phosphatase and ALT should also be monitored at week 1, week 3 and then monthly after initiation of treatment and after any increase in dose.

Stop treatment or consult rheumatologist
- total WCC <3.5 × 10⁹/l
- or neutrophil count <2 × 10⁹/l

- or platelets <140 × 10⁹/l
- if serum creatinine increases to more than 30% of baseline measurement or eGFR <45, reduce or stop treatment and discuss with rheumatologist
- 2 plusses of proteinuria
- if ALT rises more than 3 times normal, recheck after 72 hours and STOP treatment if still 3 times normal upper limit
- if ALT 2–3 times upper limit of normal, recheck after 72 hours and if still 2–3 times upper limit, reduce dosage and recheck ALT every 2 weeks
- if ALT less than twice the upper limit of normal, recheck every 2 weeks and expect to normalise in time.

Chapter 5

Biochemistry

LIVER FUNCTION TESTS (LFTs)
Serum bilirubin

- Normal range (µmol/l) is <17; total bilirubin is 3–20; indirect bilirubin is 0–14.

- Jaundice is usually only apparent with bilirubin >35.

- If serum bilirubin is elevated, check for urinary bilirubin and urobilinogen, and if LFTs are otherwise normal, ask the laboratory to specify the level of conjugated/unconjugated bilirubin (direct/ indirect).

- Normal urinary bilirubin and raised urobilinogen, in the presence of jaundice suggests haemolytic jaundice.

- Raised urinary bilirubin and absent urobilinogen in the presence of jaundice indicates obstructive jaundice.

- If haemolysis is suspected, check serum haptoglobin (normal range 500–1900 mg/l is decreased in haemolysis).

- Normal liver enzymes and normal haptoglobin exclude hepatitis and haemolytic disease.

Precautions
- Protect the sample of blood from sunlight, as light will reduce the bilirubin content.

- To prevent haemolysis, do not shake the tube containing the blood.

- Full protective measures should be adhered to in order to avoid self-contamination.

Abnormal test results

- Raised total bilirubin may be caused by hepatitis, biliary stasis, haemolysis, resolution of large haematoma or congenital causes.

- A raised level of unconjugated bilirubin suggests:

  - Gilbert's syndrome (which affects 4% of the population)

  - haemolysis (which can be confirmed by lowered haemoglobin (Hb), raised reticulocytes (>2%), reduced serum haptoglobin and increased urobilinogen present in the urine)

  - postviral hepatitis

  - mild chronic hepatitis

  - Crigler–Najjar syndrome (>85 µmol/l).

- A raised level of conjugated bilirubin (>10) suggests obstructive jaundice that may be due to:

  - liver disease

  - pancreatic disease

  - Dublin–Johnson syndrome.

Urinary bile pigments

- Bile, which is formed mostly from conjugated bilirubin, reaches the duodenum where the intestinal bacteria convert the bilirubin to urobilinogen. Most of the urobilinogen is excreted in the faeces, a large amount is transported to the liver via the circulation where it is reprocessed to bile, and the remainder (approximately 1%) is excreted by the kidneys in the urine.

- The urobilinogen test is a very sensitive way to determine liver damage, haemolytic disease and severe infections.

- In early hepatitis, mild liver cell damage or mild toxic injury, the urine urobilinogen level will increase despite an unchanged serum bilirubin level. The urobilinogen level in severe liver damage will decrease because the liver is unable to conjugate bilirubin or produce bile.

- Normal or raised bilirubin and normal or raised urobilinogen suggests hepatocellular failure.

- Normal urinary bilirubin and raised urobilinogen suggests haemolytic jaundice.

- Urine does not normally contain unconjugated bilirubin (which is not water-soluble). Raised urinary bilirubin and absent urobilinogen indicates obstructive jaundice.

- False-positive tests for urinary bilirubin may occur if the patient is taking phenothiazines.

- False-negative tests for urinary bilirubin may occur if the patient is taking rifampicin.

- If clinical jaundice is present, the serum bilirubin level is normal and bilirubin is absent from the urine, this is due to:

  - hypervitaminosis A

  - high serum carotene levels (normal range (μmol/l) is 0.7–3.7) due to excessive ingestion of carrots or pumpkins.

FAECAL UROBILINOGEN

- This compound gives the stool its brown colour.

- It is produced in the small intestine by the action of intestinal bacteria on bilirubin in the bile.

- The normal range (mg urobilinogen/g stool) is 75–350.

Factors that affect laboratory results
- Antibiotics which interfere with the growth of the bacteria necessary for the production of urobilinogen.

Abnormal test results
- Increased faecal urobilinogen levels are found in increased haemolysis of red blood cells.

- Decreased faecal urobilinogen levels are indicative of obstructive biliary disease (stools will be clay-coloured).

Jaundice

- This is usually clinically obvious when bilirubin is >35 μmol/l.

- The following points in the history may be helpful:

  - prodromal flu-like illness suggests hepatitis

  - sudden-onset jaundice with severe pain in an otherwise healthy individual suggests gallstones

  - slow development of jaundice, in the absence of pain or with dull, central abdominal pain, anorexia and weight loss, suggests carcinoma

  - previous history of hepatitis may suggest chronic active hepatitis

  - previous biliary surgery may suggest the presence of stones left in the common biliary duct

  - previous malignancy, especially of breast or bowel, may suggest a biliary secondary

  - details of alcohol intake should be sought

  - members of medical and paramedical professions are at increased risk of contracting viral hepatitis

  - foreign travel increases the risks of contracting hepatitis A or B.

- Drugs that are contraindicated and associated with jaundice include:

  - amitriptyline

  - chlorpromazine and other phenothiazines

  - chlorpropamide

  - erythromycin

  - halothane

  - imipramine

  - indomethacin

  - isoniazid

  - methyldopa

  - phenelzine

- sulphate and other monoamine oxidase inhibitors

- oral contraceptive pill

- rifampicin

- salicylates

- sulphonamides

- testosterone (some preparations only)

- thiouracil.

Alkaline phosphatase (ALP)

- The normal range (IU/l) is 90–300 (the level is dependent on the method of assay).

- Haemolysis of the blood sample may falsely lower the ALP.

- ALP is primarily produced by liver and bone (it is also produced in the placenta and gut). Raised ALP and raised gamma-glutamyl transferase (GGT) or other liver enzymes suggest cholestasis or hepatic cell damage or congestion.

- In mild liver disease (mild liver cell damage), ALP may be only slightly elevated. In acute liver disease, ALP can be markedly elevated. Once the acute phase has resolved, the ALP level very quickly decreases.

- The commonest forms of liver disease that give rise to a raised ALP are bile duct obstruction due to gallstones or pancreatic cancer, pregnancy, drugs and primary biliary cirrhosis.

- Abdominal ultrasound examination will identify gallstones, otherwise a liver screen should be performed (*see* investigation of abnormal LFTs, p. 114).

- A slightly raised ALP level is a common laboratory finding. If the test is repeated and the level continues to rise, further investigations should be performed.

- In the case of bone disorders, the ALP level is increased because of abnormal osteoblastic (cell) activity (*see* Table 5.1).

- In children, levels are 2–3 times higher than normal values in adults. During the pubertal growth spurt, levels may be even higher than this.

- In the third trimester of pregnancy, levels are high (two- to threefold).

- Post-menopausal levels are raised (if significantly raised, check GGT and other liver enzymes to determine whether hepatic cause is likely).

- Post-bony fracture levels are raised.

- An individual's ALP level remains remarkably constant up to 60 years of age.

- Paget's disease as a cause would be detected with plain X-rays or a bone scan.

- Hyperthyroidism can cause a raised ALP.

- If doubt persists about the origin of the raised ALP, this can be resolved by serum electrophoresis of the isoenzymes.

- Measurement of 5-nucleotidase (normal range 3.5–11 IU/l) can confirm or exclude hepatic origin in the presence of isolated raised ALP.

- Raised ALP and raised 5-nucleotidase suggest hepatic origin.

- Normal 5-nucleotidase excludes hepatic disease.

Abnormal test results

- ALP may be raised in hyperthyroidism (raised thyroid-stimulating hormone (TSH)).

- Raised ALP may indicate:

  - bone disease – osteomalacia and rickets (Ca^{2+} <2.12 mmol/l) primary hyperparathyroidism with bone disease (Ca^{2+} >2.65 mmol/l) or secondary hyperparathyroidism Paget's disease of the bone (alkaline phosphatase level very high) secondary carcinoma of bone (raised Ca^{2+}) myositis ossificans, *or*

  - liver disease – intra- or extrahepatic cholestasis space-occupying lesions (GGT is usually raised, but bilirubin may be normal), hepatocellular disease, *or*

  - hypo- or hyperparathyroidism (*see* p. 139).

TABLE 5.1 Biochemical findings in bone disease

	Calcium	Phosphate	Alkaline phosphatase
Osteoporosis	Normal	Normal	Normal
Osteomalacia	Normal or decreased	Normal or decreased	Increased
Paget's disease	Normal	Normal	Increased
Hyperparathyroidism	Increased	Decreased	Increased
Multiple myeloma	Normal or increased	Decreased or normal	Normal or increased

Aspartate aminotransferase (AST) and alanine aminotransferase (ALT)

- Normal range (IU/l):

  - AST <50

  - ALT <45.

- AST (previously known as serum glutamic oxalo-acetic transaminase) is not included in the LFT profile in some laboratories.

- AST is present in high concentrations in heart, liver, kidney, skeletal muscle and red blood cells.

- ALT (previously known as serum glutamic pyruvic transaminase) is present in high concentrations in the liver. It is also present in heart and skeletal muscle, but in much lower concentrations. Therefore ALT is much more specific to liver disease than is AST.

- Transaminases are usually very high in hepatocellular disease such as viral hepatitis, and are more modestly raised in chronic hepatocellular damage and obstruction.

- AST is raised in shock, whereas there is not much elevation of ALT unless liver disease is present.

- REFER patients with high ALT (e.g. >250) immediately.

- Otherwise, a moderately raised ALT is likely to be due to obesity drugs, thyroid disease, new diabetes or heart failure.

Abnormal test results

- AST levels are markedly raised after:
  - myocardial infarction (MI)
  - cardiac surgery.
- AST levels are raised in:
  - viral or toxic hepatitis
  - malignancy
  - some skeletal muscle diseases
  - trauma.
- Raised ALT, in the presence of raised ALP and with signs or symptoms of liver disease such as spider naevi, palmar erythema, hepatosplenomegaly, bruising or gynaecomastia: REFER IMMEDIATELY.
- Raised ALT – consider:
  - obesity
  - diabetes
  - thyroid disease
  - drugs, especially statins, some antibiotics, non-steroidal anti-inflammatory drugs (NSAIDs) and sulphonylureas, e.g. glibenclamide, gliclazide, glimepiride, glipizide, gliquidone and tolbutamide.
- Senna, some herbal remedies and some illicit drugs such as ecstasy can also cause an isolated raised ALT.
- Small rises in ALT are often seen after initiation of statins and often return to normal.
- If ALT is three times the upper range of normal after initiation of statin, STOP STATIN.
- ALT up to twice the normal limit, assess patient for signs of liver disease AND risk factors; repeat LFTs in 3 months and refer if ALT remains high.
- ALT is low in:
  - renal failure
  - vitamin B_6 deficiency.

GGT

- Normal range (IU/l):
  - males up to 70
  - females up to 40.
- Synthesis of GGT is stimulated by many drugs (e.g. phenytoin, phenobarbitone, primidone, alcohol and possibly some antidepressants).
- GGT is a sensitive test for excess alcohol intake, but is not specific.

Abnormal test results

- Raised GGT and raised mean corpuscular volume (MCV) suggest alcohol abuse.
- Raised GGT, history of excessive alcohol intake, raised ALT and raised MCV suggest liver cell damage.
- Very high GGT (10 times normal upper limit) occurs in biliary obstruction and hepatic malignancies.
- Raised GGT and raised ALP (more than three times upper limit of normal) suggest cholestasis.
- Raised GGT may be due to non-specific causes (e.g. MI, cerebrovascular accident, diabetes mellitus, pancreatic disease, renal failure and chronic lung disease).
- LFTs (transaminase and GGT) are also affected by lack of exercise, obesity and smoking, as well as excess alcohol intake. Elevated results may therefore occur if several of these factors coexist, even if alcohol intake is not excessive (i.e. over 21 units).
- The effect of alcohol on GGT is complex. About 50% of people who drink alcohol to excess on a regular basis will have biochemical abnormalities, while the other 50% will not. An individual who is not overweight and not taking anticonvulsants, but who has a persistently raised GGT (>80 IU/l), may be 'underestimating' their alcohol intake. (For example, people who drink excessively but only on 1 or 2 nights a week.)

Further investigation of abnormal LFTs

- Raised ALT, in the presence of raised ALP and with signs or symptoms of liver disease such as spider naevi, palmar erythema, hepatosplenomegaly, bruising or gynaecomastia: REFER IMMEDIATELY.

- Raised ALT – consider:

  - obesity

  - diabetes

  - thyroid disease

  - drugs, especially statins, some antibiotics, NSAIDs and sulphonylureas, e.g. glibenclamide, gliclazide, glimepiride, glipizide, gliquidone and tolbutamide.

- Small rises in ALT are often seen after initiation of statins and often return to normal.

- If ALT is three times the upper range of normal after initiation of statin, STOP STATIN.

- ALT up to twice the normal limit – assess patient for signs of liver disease AND risk factors, repeat LFTs in 3 months and refer if ALT remains high.

In persistently raised transaminases (up to twice the normal range but not exceeding three times the normal range), or other abnormal LFTs, the following additional investigations may be helpful.

Investigation of abnormal LFTs

- Antimitochondrial antibodies are sensitive and specific for primary biliary cirrhosis.

- Hepatitis serology, IgG antibodies are raised in acute hepatitis:

  - hepatitis B – check for surface antigen

  - hepatitis C – check for antibodies.

- Ferritin is a useful screening test for haemochromatosis (normal ferritin excludes haemochromatosis).

- Ceruloplasmin for Wilson's disease (which causes cirrhosis and a Parkinson-like syndrome) (uncommon over the age of 50).

- ceruloplasmin is REDUCED in Wilson's disease, malnutrition and nephrotic syndrome
- ceruloplasmin is INCREASED in pregnancy, some infections, malignancy and some chronic liver disease.
- Alpha-1 antitrypsin deficiency can lead to cirrhosis (as well as emphysema).
- Immunoglobulins:
  - IgG raised in acute hepatitis (consider referral)
  - IgM raised in autoimmune disease (check international normalised ratio (INR) and refer if INR >2)
  - abdominal ultrasound for intra or extra hepatic obstruction.

Serum amylase

- Normal range (IU/l) is 70–300 (depending on the method used).
- In the appropriate clinical situation, with upper abdominal pain, vomiting and abdominal tenderness, values of >1,200 are diagnostic of acute pancreatitis.
- Raised values in the range 300–1,200 may occur in:
  - cancer of the pancreas
  - perforated duodenal ulcer
  - dissecting aortic aneurysm
  - mesenteric vascular occlusion
  - small-bowel obstruction
  - ruptured ectopic pregnancy
  - acute renal failure
  - mumps
  - salpingitis
  - liver disease.
- Below-normal levels may be found in:
  - pancreatic insufficiency
  - hepatitis
  - toxaemia of pregnancy.

Pancreolauryl test
- Done over 2 days, measuring the excretion index:

  - an excretion index of >30% indicates normal exocrine pancreatic function

  - an excretion of <20% indicates pancreatic insufficiency.

Alcohol intoxication (serum volumes) and ethanol concentrations

- Subclinical intoxication (g/l): 0–1.

- Gross intoxication (g/l): 2.

- Stupor (g/l): 3.

- The legal limit for blood alcohol while driving a motor vehicle is 80 mg%.

- The legal limit for urine alcohol while driving a motor vehicle is 107 mg%.

Albumin

- Normal range (g/l) is 30–55 (depending on the method used).

Abnormal test results
- Elevated albumin levels (rare) suggest dehydration.

- If albumin levels are lowered, check for proteinuria (e.g. nephrotic syndrome, malabsorption, chronic liver disease, preeclampsia). Albumin levels are normally lowered during the third trimester of pregnancy.

- Serum albumin, bilirubin and INR, combined, are the best tests of LIVER FUNCTION.

  NB: If albumin levels are reduced, some drugs that are usually protein-bound (e.g. phenytoin, phenobarbitone, theophylline, salicylates, penicillin, sulphonamides and warfarin), will be present in higher concentration in their free forms in the bloodstream. Therefore, toxicity may be apparent at lower drug concentrations.

- Lowered albumin also affects the serum calcium level (*see* p. 136).

Globulins

- Normal range (g/l) is 16–37.

- Globulins can be separated by electrophoresis into alpha, beta and gamma globulins, although they are rarely quantified.

- All gamma globulins are immunoglobulins; IgG represents 75% of the total.

Abnormal test results

- Lowered total globulins suggest immunodeficiency syndromes.

- Elevated total globulins suggest paraproteinaemias (e.g. myeloma or chronic liver disease).

- Raised alpha-1 globulin suggests:

  - tissue damage (e.g. chronic inflammatory conditions and malignancy)

  - oestrogen therapy.

- Lowered alpha-1 globulin suggests:

  - nephrotic syndrome.

- Raised alpha-2 globulin may suggest:

  - acute inflammatory response

  - nephrotic syndrome (together with lowered albumin and lowered gamma globulin)

  - diabetes mellitus

  - malignancy

  - cirrhosis.

- Lowered alpha-2 globulin and lowered albumin suggests:

  - liver disease

  - malabsorption.

- Haptoglobin (normal range 500–1,900 mg/l is an alpha-2 globulin that is increased in acute inflammatory conditions and decreased in haemolysis. Normal liver enzymes and normal haptoglobin exclude hepatitis and haemolytic disease.

- Increased beta globulin suggests:

  - biliary obstruction

  - nephrotic syndrome

  - iron deficiency

  - pregnancy

  - oral contraceptive pill.

Gamma globulins

- Normal range (g/l) (in adults):

  - IgA, 1.5–2.5

  - IgG, 8–18

  - IgM, 0.4–2.9.

- Gamma globulins are all antibodies, and raised levels generally occur in:

  - chronic infection

  - rheumatoid arthritis (RA) (also raised alpha-2)

  - systemic lupus erythematosus

  - liver disease

  - sarcoidosis.

- Gamma globulins are commonly requested in patients presenting with recurrent chest infections or recurrent herpes infections, and in children in whom immunodeficiency is suspected.

Factors that affect laboratory results

- Immunisations, vaccinations and toxoids administered within the last 6 months.

- Blood transfusions, tetanus, anti-tetanus and gamma globulin received in the last 6 months can affect the Ig result.

Abnormal test results

- Elevated IgM suggests:

  - primary biliary cirrhosis or chronic infection

  - RA (the IgM rheumatoid factor is positive in 80% of patients with RA. The majority of the remaining 20% have IgG and IgA rheumatoid factors, but these do not show up in the standard test for rheumatoid factor).

- Antimicrobial antibodies should also be sought in primary biliary cirrhosis.

  NB: IgM is the first immunoglobulin to appear in hepatitis A or B.

- Elevated IgA suggests:

  - cirrhosis – alcoholic and other forms

  - chronic infection

  - autoimmune disease.

- IgA deficiency is associated with mild recurrent respiratory tract infections and intestinal disease.

- Elevated IgG suggests:

  - liver disease

  - autoimmune disease

  - infections.

- Decreased IgG suggests nephrotic syndrome (also lowered alpha-2 globulin and lowered albumin).

- A homogeneous band of IgG, IgM or IgA on electrophoresis usually suggests myeloma, and is usually accompanied by an erythrocyte sedimentation rate >100.

IgE

- The normal range for non-atopic adults in the UK (kU/l) is 1–180.

Bence–Jones protein

- This does not react with Albustix.

- It is found in the urine of 50% of patients with myeloma.

- Serum free light chains (kappa and lamda) may be measured instead of Bence–Jones urinary protein.

  - kappa   normal range 3.3–19.4 mg/l

  - lamda   normal range 5.7–26.3 mg/l

  - kappa/lamda ratio   normal range 0.26–1.65

- Suspect myeloma if the following abnormalities are present

  - erythrocyte sedimentation rate >30 mm/hour

  - adjusted calcium >2.65 mmol/l (parathyroid hormone low, and no known primary cancer)

  - new case of renal impairment (chronic kidney disease (CKD) stages 3–5, i.e. estimated glomerular filtration rate (eGFR) <60)

  - serum globulins >48 g/l

  - serum globulins <19 g/l

  - anaemia for no obvious reason.

Cerebrospinal fluid electrophoresis

- This may be useful for supporting a diagnosis of multiple sclerosis suggested by raised gamma globulin and oligoclonal band not mirrored in serum.

UREA AND ELECTROLYTES

Blood urea

- The normal range is up to 8.5 mmol/l (laboratory ranges may vary).

- Blood urea and creatinine are indicators of renal function.

- Neither plasma urea nor creatinine are very sensitive indicators of renal function.

- Excretion of urea (and therefore elevation of serum urea) is decreased if vascular perfusion of the kidneys is decreased (e.g. in dehydration and congestive cardiac failure).

- Lowered urea levels occur in:
  - pregnancy
  - hepatic failure
  - nephrosis
  - diabetes insipidus.
- Raised urea levels occur in renal disease and congestive cardiac failure, which is the commonest cause of a raised serum urea concentration (while the creatinine level is likely to be normal).

Serum values for urea and electrolytes

- The following values are generally accepted as the normal range. Individual values may vary slightly from one laboratory to another.
- Normal range:
  - Na^+, 135–145 mmol/l, 135–145 mEq/l
  - K^+, 3.5–5.3 mmol/l, 3.5–5.3 mEq/l
  - Cl^-, 95–105 mmol/l, 95–105 mEq/l
  - Ca^{2+} (total), 2.1–2.65 mmol/l, 8.5–10.5 mg/100 ml
  - Ca^{2+} (ionised), 1–1.25 mmol/l, 4–5 mg/100 ml
  - urea, 3.0–8.8 mmol/l, 8.0–50 mg/100 ml
  - creatinine, 60–120 µmol/l, 0.7–1.4 mg/100 ml
  - bicarbonate, 24–32 mmol/l
  - lead (red blood cell count), 0.5–1.7 µmol/l
  - Cu^{2+}, 16–31 µmol/l, 110–200 µg/100 ml
  - Zn^{2+}, 8–23 µmol/l, 0.05–0.15 mg/100 ml
  - Mg^{2+}, 0.7–1.0 mmol/l, 1.8–2.4 mg/100 ml
  - uric acid, 0.1–0.45 mmol/l, 2–7 mg/100 ml.

Electrolyte disturbances

Sodium (Na+)

- Normal range is 135–145 mmol/l.

- Increased Na^+ is nearly always due to:
  - water loss, e.g. dehydration due to diarrhoea and vomiting or to sweating because of high temperature
  - diabetes insipidus
  - primary aldosteronism.
- In diabetes insipidus, urine osmolality is reduced (<300 mOsmol/l).
- Decreased Na^+:
  - <135 mmol/l
  - significant hyponatraemia <125 mmol/l
  - may be found in:
    - —diarrhoea and vomiting
    - —drugs (e.g. potent thiazide diuretics, angiotensin-converting enzyme (ACE) inhibitors, selective serotonin reuptake inhibitors, amiodarone, phenothiazines, chlorpromazine, tricyclics, carbamazepine, cortisone preparations, desmopressin, ecstasy)
    - —heart failure (on diuretics)
    - —liver failure
    - —kidney failure (occasionally)
    - —Addison's disease (check serum cortisol at 9 a.m. – *see* p. 133)
    - —hypothyroidism
    - —alcoholism.
- SIADH (syndrome of inappropriate antidiuretic hormone) which may be caused by:
  - neurological and psychiatric disorders
  - ectopic production, e.g. small cell carcinoma lung cancer
  - lung disease
  - drugs, e.g. opiate analgesics, carbamazepine, selective serotonin reuptake inhibitors.

- Pseudohyponatraemia may be caused by:
  - hyperglycaemia
  - hyperlipidaemia
  - hyperproteinaemia.
- Check serum and plasma osmolality:
  - plasma osmolality   280–290 mOsmol/l
  - maximum urine osmolality   1,200 mOsmol/l
  - minimum urine osmolality   50 mOsmol/l.

Potassium (K^+)

- Normal range is 3.5–5.3 mmol/l.
- Haemolysis causes falsely raised serum potassium.
- Potassium greater than 6 mmol/l needs immediate repeat sample.
- Potassium greater than 7 mmol/l is a medical emergency and requires immediate hospital admission for assessment and treatment.
- Raised potassium can be caused by:
  - K^+-sparing diuretics such as amiloride and spironolactone
  - ACE inhibitors and angiotensin receptor blockers
  - beta-blockers
  - aspirin and NSAIDs, trimethoprim, heparin.

  NB: Raised K^+ levels are also found in Addison's disease (adrenal insufficiency), diabetic acidosis and renal tubular failure.

Where potassium is greater than 6 mmol/l, the patient needs immediate assessment and enquiry into symptoms of muscle weakness, fatigue and paraesthesia and repeat blood sample and perform ECG to identify arrhythmias and ECG changes of hyperkalaemia, including peaked T waves and widening of QRS complex.

- Decreased K^+ occurs:
  - in diarrhoea and vomiting
  - in response to certain drugs (e.g. non-K^+-sparing diuretics, steroids, carbenoxolone, insulin and high-dose penicillin)

- hypothermia

- stress.

NB: Low K+ levels (<3.5 mmol/l) should be avoided in patients who are taking digoxin, and in those with congestive cardiac failure or an existing cardiac arrhythmia or chronic liver disease.

- The clinical signs of K+ depletion include:

  - muscular weakness or paralysis and aching muscles

  - intestinal atony

  - increased sensitivity to digitalis

  - polyuria

  - polydypsia.

- ECG changes which occur as a result of low potassium include flattening and inversion of the T wave, prominent U waves and ST depression.

- In hypertension, particularly if symptoms of weakness, polyuria and polydypsia are present and K+ levels are low, consider Conn's syndrome (characterised by high urinary aldosterone and low plasma renin).

Creatinine

- Normal range is 60–120 mmol/l.

- Raised creatinine levels occur in acute or chronic obstruction anywhere in the urinary tract.

- Lowered creatinine levels occur in pregnancy.

- Creatinine is a more sensitive indicator of renal failure than urea but renal function may be reduced by up to 50% before creatinine level rises, so eGFR is now used in preference (*see* p. 128).

- A raised creatinine level indicates bilateral renal disease or disease in a single functioning kidney.

- An increase in serum creatinine up to 30% more than the pretreatment level is acceptable in the management of patients with renal disease, provided the serum creatinine does not exceed 150 µmol/l.

- Creatinine clearance (ml/min) = 140 – age × weight in kilograms × 1.23 divided by serum creatinine in μmol/l.

  NB: For women, multiply the resulting value by 0.85.

- Trimethoprim is a tubular toxin and can cause elevated creatinine and should not be used in patients with significant renal disease.
- Metformin should also be avoided in men with a serum creatinine of >150 mmol/l and in women with a serum creatinine of >140 mmol/l.

Chloride (Cl⁻)

- Increased Cl⁻ occurs in:
  - dehydration
  - severe diarrhoea
  - intestinal fistulae
  - respiratory alkalosis
  - primary hyperparathyroidism.
- Decreased Cl⁻ occurs in:
  - vomiting
  - diabetic ketosis
  - renal tubular damage
  - Addison's disease
  - respiratory acidosis.

Magnesium (Mg^{2+})

- Normal range: 0.7–1.0 mmol/l.
- Magnesium levels most important in patients taking proton pump inhibitors (PPIs) and citalopram and escitalopram.
- Hypomagnesia (<0.7 mmol/l may give rise to muscle cramps, weakness, tetany, tremor or fasciculation, as well as fatigue, loss of appetite or vomiting.
- Magnesium level <0.5, admit as medical emergency.

- Magnesium level 0.5–0.7, seek specialist advice, may need admission.

- Low levels may be found in:
  - chronic kidney disease, including dialysis.
  - drugs
    —loop diuretics

    —PPIs

    —cytotoxic drugs

    —immunosuppressant drugs

    —theophylline
  - poorly controlled diabetes
  - alcoholism

    —hyperparathyroidism

    —malabsorption including diarrhoea, inflammatory bowel disease and coeliac disease.

- Raised levels may be found in:
  - hypothyroidism
  - dehydration
  - lithium toxicity
  - Addison's disease.

Urate

- Normal range (mmol/l):
  - males, <0.42
  - females, <0.36.

- Asymptomatic hyperuricaemia does not need treatment.

- Normal uric acid level does not exclude gout.

- Gout is likely when uric acid levels are >360 µmol/l with normal GFR (i.e. raised levels expected in renal failure).

Test results

NB: Renal impairment leads to hyperuricaemia as do thiazide and loop diuretics. Haematological malignancies and cytotoxic drugs cause hyperuricaemia, which may lead to acute gout. Ciclisporin used in transplant patients also causes hyperuricaemia.

- Uric acid levels may be elevated in:
  - gout
  - psoriasis especially psoriatic arthropathy
  - haemolytic anaemia
  - leukaemia
  - polycythaemia
  - renal insufficiency
  - myeloproliferative diseases (including myeloma)
  - hypothyroidism
  - obesity
  - excessive alcohol intake.
- Dietary constituents that may raise urate levels include:
  - liver, kidney, turkey, shellfish, sardines, mackerel, herring, anchovies
  - meat extract, e.g. marmite, strawberries, fructose-containing soft drinks, alcohol – especially beer, red wine, fortified wines and spirits.
- Urate-lowering drugs should be used to lower uric acid levels in acute recurrent gout. The aim of treatment is to reduce uric acid levels to <0.30 mmol/l.
- In young patients with marked hyperuricaemia, measurement of the 24-hour urinary uric acid excretion on a low purine diet identifies stone producers.
- The relatives of such patients should also be investigated, as they are at risk of nephrolithiasis.

Acid phosphatase (total and prostatic)

- Normal range (IU/l):

  - total, <7.2

  - prostatic fraction, <2.2.

- Do not take the blood sample immediately following digital rectal examination.

- *See also* the section on prostate-specific antigen (PSA) (p. 155).

CHRONIC KIDNEY DISEASE (CKD)

- The eGFR is calculated from the patient's serum creatinine level and their age and sex.

- For African-Caribbean patients, the eGFR should be multiplied by 1.2 unless the laboratory has already done this.

- Relying on the serum creatinine alone for measuring renal function is not satisfactory because renal function can deteriorate by up to 50% before creatinine levels begin to rise.

- The eGFR is not applicable to patients with acute renal failure or to children under the age of 18 years.

- CKD is then classified according to eGFR (*see* Table 5.2).

TABLE 5.2 Chronic kidney disease stages

Stage 1	eGFR >90 ml/min	PLUS haematuria or proteinuria
Stage 2	eGFR 60–89 ml/min	PLUS haematuria or proteinuria
Stage 3	eGFR 30–59 ml/min	= moderate fall in eGFR
Stage 4	eGFR 15–29 ml/min	= severe fall in eGFR
Stage 5	eGFR <15 ml/min	= established renal failure

- Over the age of 40 years, there is a normal age-related decline in eGFR of approximately 1 ml/min/year.

- All patients with an eGFR <60 ml/min should be on a CKD register.

- All patients with CKD have an increased cardiovascular morbidity and mortality rate and should have their cardiovascular risk factors assessed and treated aggressively.

- Most patients with CKD stages 1–3 do not deteriorate rapidly into established renal failure unless they have significant proteinuria, otherwise they require annual measurement of the eGFR.

- All patients with stage 5 eGFR <15, or creatinine >400 (male) or >300 (female) should be referred IMMEDIATELY.

- All patients with stage 4 eGFR 15–29, or creatinine 200–400 (male) or 150–300 (female) whose results do not improve after a repeat sample 5 days later should be REFERRED urgently.

- Also refer significant proteinuria, i.e. albumin/creatinine ratio (ACR) >70 mg/mmol or urine protein/creatinine ratios (PCR) >100 mg/mmol.

Drugs which should be avoided or used with caution in patients with renal impairment (raised serum creatinine or lowered eGFR) are listed below.

ACE inhibitors and angiotensin receptor blockers
An increase in serum creatinine up to 30% more than the pretreatment level is acceptable in the management of patients with renal disease, provided the serum creatinine does not exceed 150 µmol/l.

Trimethoprim
- This is a tubular toxin and can cause elevations in serum creatinine and should be avoided in patients with significant renal disease.

Metformin
- Should be avoided in men with a serum creatinine above 150 µmol/l and in women with a level above 140 µmol/l.

- Typical repeat testing frequency for monitoring eGFR:

  - Stage 1 eGFR >90 but with other evidence of kidney damage, e.g. proteinuria or microscopic haematuria, repeat eGFR each 12 months

  - Stage 2 eGFR 60–89 with other evidence of kidney damage, repeat eGFR each 12 months

- Stage 3 eGFR 30–59 after repeat testing, i.e. result stable, with or without evidence of kidney damage, repeat eGFR each 6 months
- Stage 4 eGFR 15–29 after repeat testing, with or without evidence of kidney damage, repeat eGFR each 3 months
- Stage 5 eGFR <15 established renal failure, repeat eGFR each 6 weeks at least.

- eGFR <60 ml/min
  - check 3 previous creatinines or eGFRs over 90 days if possible
  - a decline is significant if >5 ml/min in 1 year or >10 ml/min in 5 years
  - repeat eGFR in 2 weeks if no previous record
  - assess clinical status, e.g. urine output and drug history
  - dip urine for blood and protein and send urine for ACR.

- Refer if eGFR <30 ml/min, refer urgently if eGFR <15 ml/min
  - decline is significant
  - ACR >30 or PCR >70
  - anaemia, Hb <11.

NSAIDs
- Avoid use if possible if renal impairment is present; stop if renal function is deteriorating.

Diuretics: loop diuretics (e.g. furosemide) and thiazide diuretics (e.g. bendroflumethazide)
- These can cause interstitial nephritis and should be avoided if possible in patients with poor renal function.
- K^+-sparing diuretics may cause hyperkalaemia and should be avoided if possible in patients with renal failure.

Tetracyclines
- Can cause deterioration in renal function and should be avoided if possible. Doxycycline or minocycline are safer alternatives.

Opioid analgesics

- Can cause more central nervous system depression in patients with renal impairment and should be avoided if possible. Other analgesics may cause analgesic renal nephropathy.

Aspirin and oral anticoagulants

- Should be avoided in severe renal impairment.

Disease-modifying anti-rheumatic drugs (DMARDs) (*see* p. 95)

- Many DMARDs affect renal function, which should be closely monitored.

Lithium

- This is nephrotoxic and should be used with caution in patients with renal impairment.

URINE BIOCHEMISTRY

Collection of timed urine specimens

- The accuracy of creatinine clearance and 24-hour urine results depends largely on the accuracy of the urine collection. This may be difficult to control for a variety of reasons, but errors often occur because of a misunderstanding by the doctor, nurse or patient with regard to the procedure for collecting the urine. Urine already in the bladder at the time of the start of the test must not be included in the collection. The procedure is as follows for a 24-hour urine collection required between 9 a.m. on Monday and 9 a.m. on Tuesday.

  - *9 a.m. on Monday*: empty bladder completely and *discard this specimen*. Then collect all urine passed until 9 a.m. Tuesday.

  - *9 a.m. Tuesday*: empty bladder completely and *add this specimen* to the collection.

- The components in a urine sample must be analysed within 1 hour of collection.

17-Oxosteroids (17-ketosteroids)
- Normal range (μmol/24 hours):
    - males 19–50 years, 28–76
    - females 19–50 years, 21–52
    - males >50 years, 17–63
    - females >50 years, 10–31.

Abnormal test results
- 17-Oxosteroids are raised in Cushing's syndrome.
- 17-Oxosteroids are lowered in Addison's disease, hypopituitarism.

17-Oxygenic steroids (17-hydroxycorticosteroids)
- Normal range (μmol/24 hours):
    - males 19–50 years, 28–70
    - females 19–50 years, 21–63
    - males >50 years, 17–52
    - females >50 years, 10–31.

Abnormal test results
- 17-Oxygenic steroids are raised in Cushing's syndrome.
- 17-Oxygenic steroids are lowered in:
    - Addison's disease
    - hypopituitarism.

Urinary free cortisol
- Normal range (nmol/24 hours):
    - males, <270
    - females, <260.

Abnormal test results

- Elevation of these levels suggests:
  - Cushing's syndrome (pituitary, adrenal or iatrogenic)
  - polycystic ovaries
  - some testicular cancers
  - adrenogenital syndrome.
- Random serum cortisol levels are of no help in the diagnosis of Cushing's syndrome, which is confirmed by a raised urinary free cortisol concentration. It is essential that a complete 24-hour collection of urine is made. There is a false-positive and false-negative rate of approximately 5%.

  NB: A low morning serum cortisol level (<50 nmol/l) after taking 1 mg of dexamethasone at midnight the previous night usually excludes Cushing's syndrome.

- False-positive results can be seen in:
  - pregnant women
  - patients with alcohol-related problems
  - obese individuals.
- Some drugs may also influence the results (e.g. oestrogens and anticonvulsants). False-negative results are rare (approximately 2% of cases).
- Short Synacthen test for Addison's disease:
  - take a basal serum cortisol level
  - administer 250 µg of Synacthen
  - measure serum cortisol 30 minutes and 60 minutes later.
- In healthy individuals, the basal plasma cortisol should exceed 170 nmol/l and rise to at least 580 nmol/l. The hypoadrenal patient is unable to raise the serum cortisol in response to Synacthen.

Urinary free catecholamines

- 24-hour urine collection:

  - noradrenaline, 0–700 nmol/24 hours

  - adrenaline, 0–200 nmol/24 hours

  - dopamine, 0–3 μmol/24 hours.

- 24-hour creatinine is often quoted as a guide to the reliability of the result. If the creatinine is low, this indicates too small a collection of urine took place and may invalidate the test result. Normal 24-hour urine creatinine is 8,800–17,000 μmol/l.

Vanillylmandelic acid (VMA)

- A 24-hour urine collection is required. Add 50 ml of 20% hydrochloric acid to the container before starting the collection. Collect three samples over 5 days. Include details of medication, especially aspirin and methyldopa.

- VMA is a metabolite of adrenaline and noradrenaline.

- Normal range is 0–40 μmol/24 hours.

Abnormal test results

- Raised VMA suggests:

  - phaeochromocytoma

  - neuroblastoma.

  NB: VMA may also be raised due to high dietary intake of caffeine, salicylate or bananas.

Homovanillic acid

- A 24-hour collection is required. Add 50 ml of 20% hydrochloric acid to the container before starting the collection. Collect three samples over 5 days. Include details of medication, specially aspirin and methyldopa.

- Normal range (adults) (μmol/24 hours) is <40.

- 5-Hydroxyindoleacetic acid 0–4 μmol/24 hours

- Normetadrenaline <4.4 μmol/24 hours excreted in urine in

hypertensive patient who generally excrete more metanephrines than healthy non-hypertensive patients.

- Other metanephrines, including noradrenaline, adrenaline, dopamine and metadrenaline, may be raised in phaeochromocytoma.

TABLE 5.3 Excretion of metabolites over 24 hours

	Mean		Range	
	SI unit	Traditional unit	SI unit	Traditional unit
Calcium	5.75 mmol	11.5 mEq	3.25–8.25 mmol	6.5–16.5 mEq
Chloride				
Men	184 mmol	184 mEq	120–140 mmol	120–140 mEq
Women	132 mmol	132 mEq		
Creatine			Up to 380 mmol	Up to 50 mg
Creatinine				
Men	15.8 mmol	1.8 g	9.7–23.0 mmol	1.1–2.5 g
Women	10.3 mmol	1.17 g	9.0–11.7 mmol	1.0–1.3 g
Magnesium	5.3 mmol	10.5 mEq	2.5–8.0 mmol	5.0–16 mEq
Nitrogen (total)	0.8 mmol	11.5 g	0.5–1.2 mmol	7–16 g
Oxosteroids				
Men	71 μmol	20.5 mg	59–83 μmol	17–24 mg
Women	49 μmol	14 mg	28–70 μmol	8–20 mg
Phosphate	44 mmol	1.4 g	25–62 mmol	0.8–2.0 g
Potassium				
Men	57 mmol	57 mEq	35–80 mmol	35–80 mEq
Women	47 mmol	47 mEq		
Protein		100 mg		
Sodium				
Men	177 mmol	177 mEq	120–220 mmol	120–220 mEq
Women	128 mmol	128 mEq		
Urate	3.2 mmol	0.5 g	0.5–5.9 mmol	0.1–1.0 g
Urea	342 mmol	20.6 g	209–475 mmol	12.6–28.6 g

Abnormal test results
- Raised homovanillic acid suggests:
  - phaeochromocytoma
  - neuroblastoma.

NB: Other features of phaeochromocytoma include severe hypertension, mild hyperkalaemia, raised haematocrit and impaired glucose tolerance.

5-Hydroxyindole acetic acid (5HIAA)
- Normal range (μmol/24 hours) is <31 (2–10 mg/24 hours).
- 5HIAA is a tryptophan metabolite.

Abnormal test results
- 5HIAA levels are raised in:
  - carcinoid syndrome
  - malabsorption, especially sprue and gluten intolerance.

Serum aldosterone
- Normal range (pg/ml):
  - early morning (recumbent), 12–150
  - daytime (ambulatory), 70–350.
- It is useful in testing for Conn's syndrome.

Calcium (Ca^{2+})
- Serum Ca^{2+} is a balance between Ca^{2+} absorption and renal excretion, bone resorption and bone mineralisation.
- Serum Ca^{2+} is usually expressed as protein (albumin) adjusted values, as it is about 50% bound.
- The corrected calcium concentration is the total concentration as if the albumin concentration was normal (i.e. 40 g/l).
- For every 1 g/l that the albumin concentration is below 40 g/l, the calcium concentration is 0.02 mmol/l below what it would be if the albumin concentration was normal; if the albumin is low

the corrected calcium will be actually higher than the measured calcium:

- corrected [Ca] = measured [Ca] + {(40 − [albumin]) × 0.02}.

Abnormal test results

- Ca^{2+} >2.65 mmol/l, or >2.70 mmol/l in women over 70 years of age suggests hypercalcaemia.

Hypercalcaemia

- Symptoms due to hypercalcaemia are not usually apparent until the serum Ca^{2+} is >3.0 mmol/l, when anorexia, nausea, vomiting, constipation, fatigue, weakness, depression, polyuria, polydypsia, renal colic, bone pain and pancreatitis may be features. Calcium greater than 3 mmol/l require urgent secondary investigation.

- Drowsiness and confusion are late and serious signs of hypercalcaemia.

- At >3.7 mmol/l, cardiac complications can be fatal.

- The main causes of hypercalcaemia are:
  - primary hyperparathyroidism (phosphate is usually <0.75 mmol/l), raised parathyroid hormone usually >30 ng/l
  - malignancy including bronchus, breast, genito-urinary system, squamous carcinoma of head, neck or oesophagus, multiple myeloma, lymphoma, secondary bone tumours and haematological malignancy.
  - hyperthyroidism
  - drugs including lithium and thiazide diueretics.

- Ca^{2+} <2.12 mmol/l suggests hypocalcaemia.

- Hypocalcaemia can be due to:
  - hypoparathyroidism (raised phosphate)
  - rickets
  - osteomalacia
  - chronic renal failure

- malabsorption

- nephrotic syndrome.

- Malabsorption is unlikely where there is a normal serum calcium and normal haemoglobin.

- Clinical situations in which hypercalcaemia should be considered include:

  - renal stones

  - sarcoidosis

  - toxic confusional states

  - renal failure (may cause hypocalcaemia)

  - patients taking large doses of vitamin D.

Diet in the prevention of kidney stones

- Patients with renal calculi should be advised to:

  - increase their daily fluid intake

  - reduce food high in oxalate, such as chocolate, nuts, beans, spinach and black tea

  - INCREASE rather than decrease the daily intake of calcium.

Phosphate

- Levels of phosphate are closely linked to those of Ca^{2+}.

- Normal range (mmol/l) is 0.8–1.45.

Procedure

- The patient may drink water and take their medication as usual.

- The patient should not eat for at least 8 hours before the blood sample is taken.

- The patient should not eat food with a high fat content for at least 24 hours before the test.

Factors that affect laboratory results

- A diet high in fat.

Abnormal test results
- Raised phosphate levels suggest:
  - renal failure
  - hypoparathyroidism
  - vitamin D excess.
- Lowered phosphate levels suggest:
  - hyperparathyroidism
  - rickets (except in renal failure)
  - vitamin D deficiency
  - renal tubular disease
  - bacterial septicaemia
  - insulin therapy.

NB: Drugs that can lower phosphate levels include aluminium hydroxide, anabolic steroids, oestrogen therapy and IV infusions (see also alkaline phosphatase, LFTs, p. 109).

Differential diagnosis in bone disease
- Very high alkaline phosphatase and raised Ca^{2+} suggests Paget's disease.
- Low or normal Ca^{2+} and low phosphate suggests:
  - rickets
  - osteomalacia.
- High Ca^{2+}, low phosphate, possible raised alkaline phosphatase and 'pepperpot' skull on X-ray suggests hyperparathyroidism.
- Normal alkaline phosphatase makes bony secondaries unlikely.

NB: With osteoporosis there are no biochemical changes, i.e. serum Ca^{2+} (when corrected for serum albumin) and bony alkaline phosphatase are usually normal.

Investigations for suspected primary hyperparathyroidism
- Fasting serum Ca^{2+} on 3 consecutive days, without the use of a tourniquet.

- Ca^{2+} excretion in the urine.

- Plasma phosphate.

- Parathyroid hormone assay, using a plastic syringe and plastic heparinised tube kept on ice, and centrifuging the sample immediately.

- Plain X-ray of hands and skull may show subperiosteal erosions and 'pepperpot' skull.

Blood gases (arterial)
- pH   7.36–7.44

- pO_2 11–13 kPa

- pCO_2 4.6–5.9 kPa

- HCO_3 22–26 mmol/l

    High in metabolic alkalosis and compensated respiratory acidosis
    Low in metabolic acidosis and compensated respiratory alkalosis
- O_2 saturation 95–97%

BLOOD SUGAR
- Normal range (mmol/l):

    - fasting, 3.5–5.5 (may be higher in the elderly)

    - post-prandial, up to 7.7.

- Use fluoride oxalate tubes for collection only, and store specimens in a refrigerator if there is a delay in reaching the laboratory.

- Glucose homoeostasis varies with age, sex, time of day and stage of the menstrual cycle in women.

- A *fasting* venous plasma glucose of 6.0 mmol/l or lower excludes the diagnosis of diabetes.

- A *fasting* venous plasma glucose of 6.1–6.9 mmol/l suggests *impaired glucose tolerance*, with an increased risk of developing diabetes, and a 40% greater risk of death from cardiovascular disease than people with a normal glucose tolerance. An oral glucose tolerance test is therefore recommended with periodic monitoring of blood glucose levels.

- A *fasting* venous plasma glucose of >6.9 mmol/l, with symptoms of diabetes (polyuria, polydypsia and weight loss), is diagnostic of diabetes.

- A *random, non-fasting* glucose <7.7 mmol/l excludes diabetes, >7.8 mmol/l requires further investigation with a glucose tolerance test.

- A *random* glucose of >11 mmol/l, with symptoms of diabetes (polyuria, polydypsia and weight loss), is diagnostic of diabetes.

- Patients who have no symptoms of diabetes but have a fasting venous plasma glucose >6.9 mmol/l *and* a random venous plasma of >11.0 mmol/l have diabetes mellitus.

Modified glucose tolerance test

- Patient to maintain a normal diet for 2 days.

- Patient to fast from midnight.

- At 8 a.m. ask the patient to drink ¾ pint Lucozade® within 10 minutes.

- At 10 a.m. take blood for glucose analysis.

Abnormal test results

- Normal fasting glucose <6 mmol/l and 2-hour glucose <7.8 mmol/l is normal glucose tolerance.

- Fasting glucose <7, 2-hour glucose >8 but <11 suggests impaired glucose tolerance. Check blood lipids in these patients.

- A 2-hour glucose <8 excludes diabetes.

- Fasting glucose >7, 2-hour glucose >11, confirms diabetes mellitus.

Glucose tolerance test in pregnancy

A glucose tolerance test is indicated if:
- the random plasma glucose concentration is ≥6 but ≤11 mmol/l

- there is a strong clinical indication of the possibility of gestational diabetes mellitus (GDM).

Interpretation

TABLE 5.4 Interpretation of the 75 g oral glucose tolerance test during pregnancy

Fasting glucose (mmol/l)		2-hour glucose (mmol/l)	Diagnosis	Action
≤5.5		<7.8	Normal	None
5.6–6.0	and/or	7.8–8.2	'Borderline' (gestational diabetes but low risk)	Discuss with obstetrician
>6.0	and/or	>8.2	Gestational diabetes	Refer immediately

Causes of hyperglycaemia

- Diabetes.

- Other causes of hyperglycaemia:

  - hepatic disease

  - acromegaly

  - Cushing's syndrome

  - pancreatitis

  - phaeochromocytoma

  - thyrotoxicosis

  - hyperpituitarism.

- Drugs that can cause hyperglycaemia:

  - thiazide diuretics, especially in combination with antihypertensives

  - caffeine

  - chlorpromazine

  - dexamethasone, hydrocortisone

  - oral contraceptives

  - nicotine

  - phenytoin

  - prednisolone

- probenecid

- warfarin.

Causes of hypoglycaemia

- Blood specimens transported to the laboratory in containers without preservative.

- Excess insulin or oral hypoglycaemic drug dosage in known diabetics.

- Liver failure.

- Pancreatic cell hyperplasia.

- Post-gastrectomy dumping syndrome.

- Renal failure.

- Insulinoma.

- Drugs that can cause hypoglycaemia:

  - alcohol

  - aspirin

  - barbiturates

  - beta-blockers

  - chlorpropamide

  - glibenclamide

  - insulin (overdose)

  - monoamine oxidase inhibitors

  - sulphonamides.

HbA_{1c}

- HbA_{1c} may be used to monitor the control of diabetes or is increasingly being used as a screening test for diabetes.

- Apart from diabetes, HbA_{1c} may be high in Cushing's syndrome, hyperthyroidism, phaeochromocytome, acromegaly, alcoholism and in patients who have had a splenectomy.

- HbA$_{1c}$ may be low in chronic renal failure, blood loss, haemolytic anaemia and haemoglobinopathies.

Diagnosis of diabetes using HbA$_{1c}$

- If patient has symptoms of diabetes (polydipsia, polyuria and weight loss), do NOT use HbA$_{1c}$ to diagnose diabetes but use fasting plasma glucose (>7 mmol/l) or random plasma glucose (11.1 mmol/l).
- Do NOT use HbA$_{1c}$ to diagnose diabetes in pregnancy (use fasting plasma glucose or oral glucose tolerance test).
- Do NOT use HbA$_{1c}$ to diagnose diabetes in CKD stage 4 or 5, anaemia, recent blood loss, liver disease, B$_{12}$ or folate deficiency, alcoholism, HIV or cancer treatment.
- In other random screening for diabetes, HbA$_{1c}$ >6.5% suggests diabetes but should be confirmed by a second test.
  - HbA$_{1c}$ 6–6.4% is an intermediate result and should be repeated or perform an oral glucose tolerance test
  - HbA$_{1c}$ <6 is a normal (non-diabetic) result.

Monitoring long-term control of diabetes with HbA$_{1c}$

- Guidelines:
  - overtreatment, <6
  - very good control, 6–8
  - good control, 8–9.5
  - increased therapy needed, 9.5–12
  - careful monitoring and change of therapy, >12.
- During pregnancy, a figure of <8.5 is the goal.
- HbA$_{1C}$:
  - normal, <6.5
  - acceptable, 6.5–7.5
  - high risk, >7.5.
- In the elderly, a figure of <11 is acceptable.

  NB: Local figures for these guidelines should be sought.

Target for good control of type-2 diabetes

- HbA_{1C} <7%

- Fasting plasma glucose   <6.0 mmol/l

- Blood pressure   <140/80 mmHg

- Total cholesterol   <4.8 mmol/l

- High-density lipoprotein (HDL) cholesterol   >1.2 mmol/l

- Low-density lipoprotein (LDL) cholesterol   <3.0 mmol/l

- Fasting triglyceride   <1.7 mmol/l

Serum fructosamine (mmol/l)

- Use of the fructosamine assay has replaced that of HbA_{1C} (in some laboratories) for monitoring the control of diabetes, because it is less expensive and it reflects average blood glucose levels over the preceding 2 weeks.

- Guidelines for adult diabetics:

  - good control, <2.7 mmol/l (<350 mg%)

  - control could be improved, 2.7–3.5 mmol/l (350–480 mg%)

  - poor control, >3.5 mmol/l (>480 mg%).

  NB: These ranges are only correct when the albumin concentration is normal (30–45 g/l). Figures will vary between individual laboratories.

Microalbuminuria

- A random urine sample, a timed 3-hour overnight or 24-hour urine collection, together with details of the total volume of urine, can detect microalbuminuria before proteinuria is detected on a dipstick.

Plasma insulin

- Normal range (mIU/l):

  - fasting, <19 (<0.9 µg/l)

  - 1 hour after 75 g of glucose, 50–130

  - 2 hours after 75 g of glucose, <100.

- Raised levels, in the presence of hypoglycaemia, may be due to insulinoma.

Blood ketones

Exact guidelines on the interpretation and response to blood beta-hydroxybutyrate levels are not yet established, but in the meantime, as a guide, *see* Table 5.5.

TABLE 5.5 Blood ketone levels

Blood ketone level	Recommendation
<0.6 mmol/l	No action required
0.6–1.5 mmol/l	Retest blood glucose and ketones in 2–4 hours
1.5–3.0 mmol/l	'At risk' of diabetic ketoacidosis
>3.0 mmol/l	Immediate emergency care of diabetes required

Blood homocysteine levels

- Normal range: 4–15 µmol/l.

- Elevated blood homocysteine level is an independent risk factor for cardiovascular disease, though raised homocysteine levels do not cause added risk but indicate an already existing risk.

- Raised blood homocysteine levels are common in the general population.

- Lowering homocysteine levels by taking B vitamins and folic acid does not reduce cardiovascular risk and may even increase the risk of adverse cardiovascular events.

- Patients with Alzheimer's disease and vascular dementia frequently have high homocysteine levels. Homocysteine levels are a risk factor for developing dementia.

- Patients with high homocysteine levels often have a high MCV and often have folate or B_{12} deficiency, which should be measured and treated appropriately.

- Patients with established dementia should have B_{12} and folate levels checked periodically.

Growth hormone

- Serum insulin-like growth factor-1 (IGF-1) level is age related, but levels <0.8 mU/l exclude acromegaly.

- Acromegaly is caused by excess growth hormone, usually from a pituitary adenoma.

- Symptoms (enlarged hands, feet and jaw, excess tiredness, snoring, hyperhidrosis, hypertension, diabetes) usually appear in adults between ages 30 and 50 years.

- Patients with suspected acromegaly should be referred to an endocrinologist.

- The diagnosis of acromegaly is confirmed by IGF-1 level outside the normal age/sex range AND failure of the IGF-1 level to suppress to <1 mU/l following a 75 g oral glucose tolerance test.

CARDIAC TROPONINS

- As well as creatine kinase (CK) and its MB isoenzyme (CK-MB), troponin T and troponin I can be measured to detect cardiac muscle damage. Troponin C is present in and released by skeletal muscle following damage.

- Cardiac troponin T and I are the principal test used in diagnosing acute cardiac muscle damage.

- Reference ranges vary from laboratory to laboratory and will be quoted with results.

- Troponin T and troponin I levels rise 3–6 hours after cardiac damage and reach a peak about 20 hours after cardiac damage.

- Levels remain elevated for up to 10 days following cardiac damage.

- Blood should ideally be taken 6–9 hours after the onset of chest pain and, if possible, should also be measured 12–24 hours after the onset of chest pain.

- Although elevated levels of troponin T or troponin I indicate cardiac muscle damage, this may be caused by pathologies other than acute myocardial infarction such as:

  - myocarditis

- trauma to cardiac muscle such as following a road traffic accident

- heart failure

- cardiac damage following pulmonary embolism

- cardiac damage following acute coronary artery spasm following use of cocaine.

- Levels can also be raised in renal failure but will remain constant and show no change if the sample is repeated.

- Higher levels of cardiac troponin are indicative of more severe cardiac damage.

CREATINE KINASE (CK)

- CK is most commonly checked in patients with myalgia, particularly patients who report myalgia while taking statins.

- Myalgia is more likely in older patients, those with CKD and those with a high alcohol intake.

- Myalgia can also occur in hypothyroidism, polymyalgia rheumatic (PMR) and polymyositis.

- Statins and drugs that inter-react with statins, including calcium channel blockers, macrolides and grapefruit juice, may all increase the risk of myalgia.

- CK >10 times upper limit of normal laboratory value, STOP statin immediately and check urine for blood, which can indicate rhabdomyolysis.

- CK >5 times upper limit of normal, STOP statin.

- CK <5 times the upper limit of normal, no action usually required, although consider reducing dose of statin or switch to another statin or another lipid-lowering agent if myalgia persists.

LACTIC DEHYDROGENASE (LDH)

- LDH is present in the heart, skeletal muscle, liver, kidney, brain and red blood cells.

- Five isoenzymes exist. The heart principally contains LDH_1, and the liver and skeletal muscle contain primarily LDH_4 and LDH_5.

- The normal range (IU/l) is 100–500.

Abnormal test results

- Elevated LDH suggests acute MI, if the patient's history is suggestive.

- CK is more valuable in the first 48 hours.

NB: Elevation of other isoenzymes (<5% of results) occurs in haemolysis, megaloblastic anaemia, leukaemia, liver disease, hepatic congestion, renal disease, some neoplasms, pulmonary embolism, myocarditis, skeletal muscle disease and shock. They are also raised in haemolysed blood samples and following paracetamol overdose.

TABLE 5.6 Cardiac enzymes following MI

	Onset of rise (hours)	Peak (hours)	Duration or rise (days)
Enzyme			
CK	4–8	24–48	3–5
LDH	12–24	48–72	7–12

THYROID FUNCTION TESTS (TFTs)

- Normal range (serum values):
  - total thyroxine (T_4), 60–135 nmol/l
  - tri-iodothyronine (T_3), 1.1–2.8 nmol/l
  - TSH, 0.3–5.5 mIU/l
  - serum free T_4, 9.4–25 pmol/l
  - thyroid peroxidase antibodies, up to 35 kU/l
  - serum free T_3, 3.0–8.6 pmol/l
  - thyroxine-binding globulin (TBG), 8–15 mg/l, T_4 / TBG ratio, 6:12.

Abnormal test results

- Raised serum T_4 occurs in:

  - thyrotoxicosis

  - oestrogen therapy and during pregnancy

  - liver disease

  - porphyria

  - familial TBG excess

  - drugs (e.g. thyroxine, amiodarone, propranolol, amphetamines, heparin).

- Lowered serum T_4 occurs in:

  - myxoedema

  - nephrotic syndrome

  - hepatic failure (due to lowered serum albumin)

  - kidney failure

  - Cushing's syndrome

  - congenital TBG deficiency

  - hypopituitarism

  - drugs (e.g. phenytoin, NSAIDs).

TSH

- A very low TSH (<0.03) is indicative of hyperthyroidism. A TSH of 0.03–0.5 is suggestive of hyperthyroidism and indicates that full TFTs are necessary.

- Low TSH suggests:

  - thyrotoxicosis

  - overtreatment with thyroxine of an underactive gland.

- Raised T_4, raised T_3 and lowered TSH suggests thyrotoxicosis.

- If the result is borderline, repeat the test in 3 months.

- Other laboratory tests in hyperthyroidism may show:

  - mild hypercalcaemia

  - mildly abnormal LFTs.

- A TSH <0.1 mIU/l is associated with a doubling of cardiovascular mortality over 10 years and a 30% 10-year risk of developing atrial fibrillation over age 60 years.

  NB: When treating thyrotoxicosis with radioactive iodine, the effect is not seen until about 6 weeks later. Following treatment with radioactive iodine, hypothyroidism often occurs.

When treating a patient with a history of thyroid cancer the TSH should be suppressed ideally to <0.05.

- Lowered TSH and T_4 suggests:

  - hypopituitarism

  - overtreatment with thyroxine

  - pituitary disease with or without hypothyroidism.

- Elevated TSH (>10) is diagnostic of primary hypothyroidism.

- Raised TSH suggests:

  - myxoedema

  - undertreatment with thyroxine

  - overtreatment with carbimazole or phenylthiouracil.

- If TSH is raised but <10 mmol/l, and the free T_4 is normal, repeat TSH and T_4 in 6–8 weeks and perform thyroid peroxidase (TPO) antibodies test. Consider other causes of raised TSH and normal free T_4 such as Addison's disease (low Na^+, raised K^+, raised urea, raised albumin).

- If TSH remains elevated but <10 mmol/l and TPO antibodies are detected (subclinical hypothyroidism), it is reasonable to start treatment with 25 µg thyroxine and repeat the TSH measurement in 3 months.

- If TSH is >10 mmol/l, *even with a normal TPO*, thyroxine treatment is necessary.

- Hypothyroid women on thyroxine replacement therapy and on hormone replacement therapy or the combined oral contraceptive pill may need to increase their dose of thyroxine; they should have their TFTs measured 12 weeks after commencing therapy.

- Other laboratory tests in hypothyroidism may show:

  - hyponatraemia macrocytosis with or without anaemia

  - mildly abnormal LFTs

  - raised CK.

- In treating hypothyroidism, check TFTs every 6 weeks and anticipate that patient will feel better within 3–6 months.

- Post-partum thyroiditis is common with a prevalence of 16% and classically has three phases:

  - thyrotoxic between 1–3 months post delivery

  - hypothyroid 3–6 months post delivery

  - recovery back to normal thyroid function by 12 months post delivery.

Haemagglutination tests for thyroid antibodies

- Normal range:

  - microsome titre, up to 800

  - colloid titre, up to 800 (also known as thyroglobulin antibodies).

Abnormal test results

- A value of >1600 suggests:

  - autoimmune disease (e.g. Hashimoto's disease) (levels are often very high)

  - Graves' disease

  - simple myxoedema.

Thyroid peroxidase antibodies

- Normal range is up to 35 kU/l.

- Following an autoimmune antibody assay, if thyroid antibody staining is positive, a thyroid peroxidase antibodies test may be performed.

- A high titre indicates a need for regular thyroid function testing.

Long-acting thyroid stimulator antibody
- This may be present in approximately 60% of patients with hyperthyroidism.

Thyroglobulin antibody
- This is positive in 25% of cases of hyperthyroidism and in autoimmune thyroiditis.

Anti-microsomal thyroid antibody
- This is often present in hyperthyroidism and in chronic thyroiditis.

- It is positive in Hashimoto's thyroiditis and in some cases of Graves' disease.

BLOOD LIPIDS

- Cholesterol is derived from dietary sources (a small proportion), chiefly egg yolks, offal and some seafood, but at least 50% of the body cholesterol is synthesised in the liver.

- There is a strong positive association between plasma total LDL cholesterol and the risk of coronary events.

- A reduction in total cholesterol (TC) concentration of 10% will reduce the risk of coronary heart disease (CHD) by 20%.

- Triglycerides (TGs) are the main dietary lipids found in dairy products and meat fat.

- An increase in LDL leads to hypercholesterolaemia, while an increase in very-low-density lipoprotein leads to hypertriglyceridaemia.

- LDL is the major cholesterol particle in plasma, and high levels are strongly implicated in the formation of atheroma.

- The ideal TC level recommended by the British Hyperlipidaemia Association is <5.0 mmol/l (about 80% of UK adults have TC levels of >5.3 mmol/l) and LDL <3 mmol/l.

- Haemolysis of a blood sample can falsely raise cholesterol.

- Patients at high risk should be aiming for total cholesterol <4 mmol/l and LDL <2 mmol/l or at least a 25% reduction in total cholesterol and 30% reduction on LDL.

- Day-to-day variation in TC is in the range of 4–14%. Laboratory variation may account for a further 3–5% difference in two consecutive samples. Desktop analysers may have a degree of error of up to 10%.

- Fasting is unnecessary for lipid testing. Total cholesterol and HDL are unaffected, LDL may vary by 10% and TGs may vary by 20%.

- Measure lipids 3 months after starting treatment including LFTs and CK if muscle pains occur.

LDL and HDL

- LDL = total cholesterol minus HDL minus TG/2.

- Calculation of LDL is not valid if serum triglyceride levels exceed 4.5 mmol/l.

- LDL increases with age, particularly in women, whereas HDL remains constant.

- After puberty, HDL is lower in men than in women. Oestrogens lower LDL and raise HDL.

- Blood lipids can be altered after any acute illness, including MI, and should not therefore be measured until 3 months after the event.

- Females with raised cholesterol levels are hypothyroid until proven otherwise, but renal and hepatic function and fasting blood glucose levels are also essential measurements.

- Cholesterol levels of >6.5 mmol/l approximately double the risk of CHD, and levels above 7.8 mmol/l treble it.

For the proposed Joint British Societies Cardiovascular Disease risk assessment charts (non-diabetic men and women), *see* www.bhsoc.org/files/6713/4305/2682/Proposed_Joint_British_Societies_Cardiovascular_Disease.pdf

TGs

- The relationship between raised TGs and CHD is stronger in women and in younger patients, but alcohol and diet can obscure the relationship to CHD.

- TGs >2.3 should be investigated. If TC is normal, assess other risk factors for CHD. If cholesterol levels are also elevated, look for secondary causes such as diabetes, CKD, hypothyroidism, liver disease, excess alcohol intake, and diuretic or beta-blocker therapy or oral oestrogens. Refer to lipid clinic any TG >10 (risk of pancreatitis), refer urgently if >20.

Diagnosing familial hyperlipidaemia (FH)

- FH should be diagnosed based on the Simon Broome criteria. That is, definite FH with raised TC >7.5 mmol/l or LDL >4.0 mmol/l and tendon xanthoma or evidence of FH in first- or second-degree relatives or a positive DNA test for the underlying genetic disorder or possible FH with cholesterol levels as above and a history of MI in a second-degree relative under the age of 50 years or a first-degree relative under the age of 60 years.

- In children (under 16 years) the above cholesterol measurements apply but with reduced levels of TC (>6.7 mmol/l and LDL >4 mmol/l).

- Patients with xanthelasmata are at increased risk of cardiovascular disease regardless of cholesterol levels, whereas patients with arcus corneae are at no increased risk.

Monitoring statin therapy

- LFTs (or just the ALT) are required before commencing treatment with a statin.

- Three months after commencing statin therapy, measure lipids, LFTs (ALT) and possibly creatine kinase.

- Repeat LFTs (ALT) 6-monthly or sooner if dose of statin increased.

- Stop statin if transaminase levels are 3 times the upper limit of the normal range, or if creatine is 'significantly raised', particularly if the patient complains of muscle cramps.

Prostate-specific antigen (PSA)

- PSA is a glycoprotein specific to prostatic tissue. It is regarded as a useful tool for monitoring the response to treatment of prostatic cancer, and as a predictor of relapse. It is also being increasingly used as a screening test.

- Do not perform a PSA test within 48 hours of ejaculation or vigorous exercise or within 1–4 weeks of acute urinary infection, or within 6 weeks of prostate biopsy.

- When the total PSA is raised, the free/total PSA ratio increases the specificity (i.e. there are fewer false-positives) of the test.

TABLE 5.7 PSA age reference ranges

Age (years)	Total PSA reference range (µg/l)
40–49	0–2.5
50–59	0–3.5
60–69	0–5.0
70–79	0–6.0

- When the age-specific PSA is borderline raised, check mid-stream urine specimen and treat urinary infection as appropriate and repeat PSA in 1–3 months.

- A 60-year-old man with a single PSA of <1.4 mg/l is unlikely to develop prostate cancer that will shorten his life expectancy.

- In all men with results in the range 4–9.0 µg/l, and in men under 59 years with a raised PSA (>3.5 for age 50–59 years, and >2.5 for age ≤49 years), the free/total PSA ratio may be helpful:

  - >15%, malignancy is unlikely

  - 5–15%, requires investigation

  - <5%, malignancy is more likely.

- The percentage of free PSA or free/total PSA is not reliable when the total PSA >10 mg/l.

PSA velocity
- An increase of more than 25% in the PSA level within 12 months, or an increase of >0.7 mg/l in 12 months is significant and warrants referral.

PCA3 is the most reliable blood test for prostate cancer but is not yet available as a screening test at the expense of the National Health Service.

Gleason score in prostate cancer

The Gleason grading system defines five histological patterns or grades with decreasing differentiation. The primary and secondary patterns, i.e. the most prevalent and the second most prevalent patterns, are added to obtain a Gleason score or sum.

Gleason pattern 1

- Composed of a very well-circumscribed nodule of separate, closely packed glands that do not infiltrate into adjacent benign prostatic tissue.

- Glands are of intermediate size, and similar in size and shape.

- Pattern is usually seen in transition zone cancers.

- Gleason pattern 1 is exceedingly rare.

Gleason pattern 2

- Comprising round or oval glands with smooth ends. The glands are more loosely arranged and not quite as uniform in size and shape as those of Gleason pattern 1.

- May be minimal invasion by neoplastic glands into the surrounding non-neoplastic prostatic tissue.

- Glands are of intermediate size and larger than in Gleason pattern 1.

- Variation in glandular size and separation between glands is less than that seen in pattern 3.

- Gleason pattern 2 is usually seen in transition zone cancers but may occasionally be found in the peripheral zone.

Gleason pattern 3

- The most common histological pattern.

- The glands are more infiltrative and the distance between them is more variable than in patterns 1 and 2.

- Malignant glands often infiltrate between adjacent non-neoplastic glands.

- Glands of pattern 3 vary in size and shape and are often angular.

- Small glands are typical for pattern 3, but there may also be large, irregular glands.

- Each gland has an open lumen and is circumscribed by stroma.

Gleason pattern 4

- Glands appear fused, cribriform or they may be poorly defined. Fused glands are composed of a group of glands that are no longer completely separated by stroma.

- The edge of a group of fused glands is scalloped and there are occasional thin strands of connective tissue within this group.

- The hypernephroid pattern described by Gleason is a rare variant of fused glands, with clear or very pale-staining cytoplasm.

Gleason pattern 5

- An almost complete loss of glandular lumina, with only occasional lumina apparent.

- Epithelium forms solid sheets, solid strands or single cells invading the stroma.

Gleason scores of 7–10 are associated with worse prognoses.

Gleason scores of 5 and 6 are associated with lower progression rates after definitive therapy.

Testing for *Helicobacter pylori*

- *H. pylori* is implicated in peptic ulceration, and its eradication can lead to healing of ulcers. Its relevance in non-ulcer dyspepsia is less clear.

- *H. pylori* can be detected from biopsy specimens at endoscopy, or by serology or the urea breath test. The urea breath test requires the patient to swallow a radiolabelled carbon isotope, which is exhaled as radiolabelled carbon dioxide.

- An exhaled $^{14}CO_2$ of >0.25 indicates the presence of *H. pylori*, or the failure of eradication following treatment.

- Exhaled $^{14}CO_2$ is expressed as % dose/mmol CO_2 multiplied by the patient's body weight in kilograms.

FAECAL FATS

- The test for fat in the stool is used to determine the malabsorption syndrome. Stool specimens are collected to see if fat is being digested.

- Fat will not be digested if the patient has pancreatic disease with a deficiency of lipase, biliary obstruction or some other intestinal malabsorption condition.

- If there is steatorrhoea or excess fat in the stools, the latter will be frothy, foul smelling, greyish and greasy. The patient will also have foul-smelling flatus.

- Normal range (mmol/24 hours):

  - adults, 5–18

  - children >6 years, <14.

Factors that affect the laboratory results
- Ingestion of barium will make the test invalid for 48 hours.

- Mineral oil, laxatives and enemas will interfere with testing, and should not be administered.

Test results
- Raised levels suggest:

  - malabsorption

  - pancreatic disease.

Reducing substances
- Their presence in the faeces suggests malabsorption (e.g. lactase intolerance).

COELIAC DISEASE

- Clinical features:

  - iron-deficiency anaemia

  - weight loss

  - diarrhoea or constipation

- abdominal pain

- failure to thrive (in children).

- IgA anti-gliaden antibody level raised:

  - normal, 2–90 U/l.

- Anti-endomysial antibodies also raised.

- High-risk groups of patients who should be screened for coeliac disease include:

  - patients with family history of coeliac disease (10% chance in first-degree relative)

  - patients with type 2 diabetes

  - patients with Down's syndrome (40 times greater chance)

  - patients with autoimmune thyroid disease

  - infertile couples

  - patients with unexplained anaemia, especially if resistant to oral iron

  - patients with unexplained diarrhoea and/or constipation

  - all patients with a working diagnosis of irritable bowel syndrome who have not had other investigations.

TABLE 5.8 Commonly used medications and their laboratory monitoring requirements

Drug	Monitoring	Frequency	Potential hazards
Thyroxine	TSH	4-weekly until TSH within normal range, then annually	
Lithium	Lithium levels FBC	Measure blood level 12 hours after dose	
	Urea and electrolytes plus TFTs	Measure weekly until stable (2 weeks usually), then monitor 3-monthly	
		Measure if toxicity suspected (nausea, diarrhoea, polydypsia, polyuria)	
		3- to 6-monthly when levels stable	
DMARDs, e.g. penicillamine, azathiaprine, sulphasalazine, methotrexate, hydroxychloroquine, gold and leflunomide	See separate guidelines, p. 95		
Amiodarone	LFTs, TSH	Check before treatment and then every 6 months	If hyperthyroidism or hypothyroidism develop, REFER
Thiazide and loop diuretics	Urea and electrolytes	Check before treatment, 1 month after commencement of treatment, then annually	Consider K-sparing diuretic if K <3mmol/l
			Monitor K more closely in patients taking digoxin

(continued)

Drug	Monitoring	Frequency	Potential hazards
K-sparing diuretics	Urea and electrolytes	Check before treatment, 1 month after commencement of treatment and then annually	Stop treatment if K >5.3 mmol/l
ACE inhibitors	Urea and electrolytes and eGFR	Check before treatment, 2 weeks after commencement of treatment, and then annually (more frequent unless renal impairment already exists)	Stop or reduce dose if K rises >6 mmol/l
Digoxin	Serum levels of digoxin should be measured 6 hours after last dose. Also, attention should be paid to eGFR and K levels	Before treatment and if toxicity suspected, e.g. patient confused, nauseous; visual disturbance or delirium present	Stop if toxicity suspected, reintroduce at a lower dose and add K or K-sparing diuretic
Statins	LFTs	Before treatment, after 3 months of treatment, then after 6 months, and then annually. See separate guidance on abnormal LFTs in patients taking statins, p. 155	Adjust statin dosage to achieve target. Stop if ALT > three times normal

Chapter 6

Miscellaneous

THERAPEUTIC TARGET RANGES OF COMMONLY MONITORED DRUGS

- Check local laboratory ranges.

- Write on request form stated time of the last dose.

  NB: Digoxin toxicity is normally associated with serum levels >3 ng/ml, although it can be toxic within the therapeutic range. Many patients complain of sedation at therapeutic phenobarbitone levels of >25 mg/l (100 μmol/l).

Lithium carbonate

- Therapeutic range (mmol/l): 0.4–0.8 12 hours post-ingestion.

Precautions

- Plasma concentrations must be measured regularly (every 1–3 months on stabilised regimens).

- Thyroid function must be checked regularly and adequate sodium and fluid intake maintained.

- Urea, electrolytes, creatinine and thyroid function tests should be measured annually unless indicated sooner.

Possible contraindications

- *Avoid* in renal impairment, cardiac disease, conditions with sodium imbalance, e.g. Addison's disease.

- *Caution* in pregnancy (foetal intoxication), breast-feeding mothers, elderly patients, myasthenia gravis and diuretic treatment.

TABLE 6.1 Therapeutic target range of commonly monitored dug

	Metric units	Molar units
Aminophylline	10–15 µg/ml	
Carbamazepine	4–10 mg/l	17–42 µmol/l
Clonazepam	15–60 µg/l	60–150 nmol/l
Digoxin	0.5–2.0 ng/ml	1.0–2.6 nmol/l
(assuming normal potassium and renal function)		
Digoxin toxicity is likely at levels above 3.5 nmol/l		
Ethosuxamide	40–100 mg/l	283–708 µmol/l
Isoniazid	1–7 mg/l	
Lithium	4–11 mg/l	0.4–1.2 mmol/l
Phenobarbitone	10–40 mg/l	40–172 µmol/l
Phenytoin	10–20 mg/l	40–80 µmol/l
Primidone	5–15 mg/l	23–55 µmol/l
Procainamide	4–8 µg/ml	17–34 µmol/l
Sodium valproate	50–100 mg/l	347–693 µmol/l
Theophylline	10–20 mg/l	56–111 µmol/l

Dosage

- Initially 0.25–2.0 g daily.

- Start with 200–500 mg lithium carbonate for the first week or two, measuring the serum lithium weekly and increasing the dose of lithium (Li$^+$) to between 300 and 1250 mg nocte until the serum level reaches 0.4–0.8 mmol/l.

- Adjust to achieve plasma concentration on 0.4–0.8 mmol/l by tests on samples taken 12 hours after the preceding dose on the 4th and 7th days of treatment, then weekly until dosage has remained constant for 4 weeks, and monthly thereafter.

- Daily doses are usually divided and sustained-release preparations are normally given twice daily.

- Dose adjustment may be necessary in the case of diarrhoea, vomiting and heavy sweating.

- To prevent relapse of mania and depression, serum levels of 0.4–1.0 mmol/l should be aimed for.

- For prophylaxis of bipolar depression, the ideal therapeutic range is 0.8–1.0 mmol/l.

Side effects

- Short term:
  - diarrhoea
  - fine tremor
  - indigestion
  - nausea
  - polydypsia
  - polyuria
  - fatigue.

- Long term:
  - The above plus:
    —exacerbation of psoriasis
    —hypothyroidism
    —memory loss
    —weight gain.

Overdosage

- The following *will* occur with severe Li^+ overdose, i.e. plasma concentration >2 mmol/l:
  - hyper-reflexia
  - hyperextension of limbs
  - convulsions
  - toxic psychoses
  - syncope

- oliguria
- circulatory failure
- coma.
- The following *may* occur with severe Li^+ overdose:
  - goitre
  - raised antidiuretic hormone concentration
  - hypothyroidism
  - hypokalaemia
  - ECG changes
  - exacerbation of psoriasis
  - kidney changes
  - death.

Drugs affecting Li⁺ levels

- Drugs that increase plasma Li^+:
  - phenylbutazone and possibly other non-steroidal anti-inflammatory drugs
  - thiazide diuretics, e.g. bendrofluazide (Aprinox, Centyl, Neo Naclex), chlorthalidone, xipamide (Diurexan) and indapamide (Natrilix)
  - other K^+-sparing diuretics, e.g. triamterene (Dytac) do not have any effect on serum Li^+
  - since ibuprofen is available over the counter, patients should be warned of the possible adverse effects; aspirin has no such effect.
- Drugs that decrease plasma Li^+:
  - theophylline acetazolamide
  - Sandocal
  - Fybogel
  - some antacids, e.g. sodium bicarbonate, magnesium trisilicate (Gaviscon).

NB: Cessation of Li⁺ therapy 2–3 days before elective surgery should be considered, although the risk of precipitating a psychotic relapse should be weighed against the benefits.

INTERPRETATION OF CERVICAL SMEARS

This is a guide to descriptive terminology used by laboratories when reporting cervical smears. Different laboratories may use different terms, and if there is any doubt about the meaning of a report or what action should be taken, the individual laboratory should be consulted.

Inflammatory changes

- This is a redundant term that is no longer routinely reported and has been largely replaced by 'borderline changes'.

Action

- Repeat the smear at least twice before returning to normal recall.

  NB: A negative smear with inflammatory changes does not require follow-up in the absence of the report of a specific infection, but may require further investigation if appropriate.

Dyskariosis

- Changes in squamous epithelial cells, which may indicate the presence of cervical intra-epithelial neoplasia (CIN), are reported as dyskariotic and graded 'mild', 'moderate' or 'severe' (roughly equivalent to CIN 1, CIN 2 and CIN 3, respectively).

- Severe dyskariosis may be reported as abnormal squamous cells suggesting carcinoma *in situ*.

- Human papilloma virus (HPV) infection may be indistinguishable from mild dyskariosis.

Action

- Colposcopy is necessary for all moderate and severe dyskariosis, but for mild dyskariosis a single repeat smear is usually required to confirm the diagnosis.

HPV infection

- Changes due to HPV are reported together with the nuclear abnormality, such as dyskariosis or borderline changes.

- If cytological evidence of HPV is present but there is no evidence of dyskariosis, then the smear is reported as borderline and the HPV changes are noted on the smear report.

Action

- The management of sub-clinical HPV infection is dependent on the degree of nuclear abnormality present, as is the recall of women with evidence of HPV on the cervical smear.

- HPV infection may mimic the changes of mild dyskariosis (e.g. at colposcopy, evidence of HPV Infection may be found with no evidence of CIN).

Koilocytes

- These are cells with a halo around their nucleus.

- They indicate infection with HPV, which may be involved in the aetiology of CIN.

Dyskeratosis

- There is cornification/keratinisation of cells.

- This also indicates infection with HPV.

Borderline changes

- Cells cannot be described as normal.

- Changes resembling mild dyskariosis may be present.

- In patients with persistent borderline changes, this may indicate the presence of CIN.

Action

- Follow the local laboratory guidelines.

- The usual laboratory policy is to refer for colposcopy after three borderline smear reports.

Glandular abnormalities
- Abnormal glandular cells in the cervical smear may arise from the endocervix or less often from the endometrium.

Action
- Refer the patient.

Actinomyces or *Actinomyces*-like organisms
See p. 61.

Metaplastic cells
- These are normal cells from the transformation zone.
- Occasionally atypical metaplastic cells are observed, which are likely to be due to inflammation or HPV infection. Squamous or endocervical neoplasia is less likely.

Action
- Repeat the smear and refer the patient for colposcopy if the condition is persistent.

Abnormal metaplastic cells
- These are more likely to be neoplastic, and are usually squamous rather than glandular.

Action
- Refer the patient for colposcopy.

Quality of cervical smears
- Some laboratories comment on the quality of cervical smears.
- The perfect smear should contain endocervical cells, metaplastic cells and squamous cells, all in adequate numbers (*see* the British Society for Clinical Cytology guidelines on the next page).
- Where the laboratory classifies smears as 'good', 'adequate', 'acceptable' or 'poor', a clear understanding of these terms should exist.

- 'Good' or 'adequate' indicates that there is sufficient cellular material to exclude any abnormalities requiring follow-up.

- 'Acceptable' or 'poor' will require a repeat smear sooner than 3 years, and the laboratory will usually indicate how soon this should be. An endocervical brush may be necessary for the repeat smear.

- In women using oral contraceptives, smears should be taken during the first half of the cycle, e.g. days 4–15.

- In women not using oral contraceptives, smears should be taken any time except the first 4 days.

British Society for Clinical Cytology guidelines

- The transformation zone should be the prime target for cervical cytology sampling.

- The ideal smear should contain endocervical cells, metaplastic cells, endocervical mucus and squamous cells.

- Squamous cells and at least two of the other three elements should be present in an adequate smear.

- The cells on the slide should appear to be associated together in streaks rather than having the flat, rather dispersed appearance of a vaginal smear.

- The quality of this cellular material should be such that, if condensed into an area of 40×22 mm, the epithelial cells would occupy at least 25% of this area. The quality of the material is more important than the quantity.

Postnatal smear

- Many polymorphs may be present and obscure the cells such that abnormal cells cannot be excluded.

- The smear may be affected by altered hormonal status.

Action

- The smear should be repeated.

  NB: A laboratory report of an apparently low oestrogen level may be made on a smear taken shortly after a pregnancy, or it may indicate an endocrine abnormality or exogenous hormones.

Smears following a hysterectomy

- A woman who has had normal smears and is on normal routine follow-up does not require any further smears following a hysterectomy (unless advised by the hospital following histology of the uterus).

- A woman who has never had a smear or has not been on a routine smear recall register in the past should have a vault smear 6 months post hysterectomy.

- A woman with a past history of CIN which has been complelety excised should have vault cytology 6 and 18 months post hysterectomy.

- A woman who has had incomplete or uncertain excision of CIN should have vault cytology at 6, 12 and 24 months following CIN 1 or vault cytology at 6 and 12 months followed by nine annual vault smears following CIN 2/3.

CA 125

- The measurement of CA 125 combined with abdominal or transvaginal ultrasound may be used for detection of ovarian cancer.

- National Institute for Health and Clinical Excellence guidelines 2011 suggest check CA 125 if a woman presents with bloating, abdominal distension or pain, increased urinary frequency or urgency, or early satiety. Suspicion of ovarian cancer should also be considered in patients over age 50 with irritable bowel syndrome and especially patients with any of the foregoing symptoms who have a positive family history of ovarian or breast cancer.

- If CA 125 >35, arrange pelvic ultrasound scan.

- In women under 40 with suspected ovarian cancer, measure levels of alpha-fetoprotein and beta-human chorionic gonadotrophin as well as serum CA 125, to help identify women with germ cell tumours.

Calculate risk of malignancy (RMI)

The Risk of Malignancy Index combines three pre-surgical features: serum CA 125 (CA 125), menopausal status (M) and ultrasound score (U). The RMI is a product of the ultrasound scan score, the menopausal status and the serum CA 125 level (IU/ml).

$$RMI = U \times M \times CA\ 125$$

The ultrasound result is scored 1 point for each of the following characteristics: multilocular cysts, solid areas, metastases, ascites and bilateral lesions. U = 0 (for an ultrasound score of 0), U = 1 (for an ultrasound score of 1), U = 3 (for an ultrasound score of 2–5).

The menopausal status is scored as 1 = pre-menopausal and 3 = post-menopausal. The classification of 'post-menopausal' is a woman who has had no period for more than 1 year or a woman over 50 who has had a hysterectomy.

Serum CA 125 is measured in IU/ml and can vary between 0 and hundreds or even thousands of units.

- RMI >200, refer.

- CA 125 can be raised in:

    - pregnancy

    - endometriosis

    - fibroids

    - other malignancies.

Endometrial cancer

The thicker the endometrium, the higher the risk of endometrial cancer. A thickness of <5 mm has a negative predictive value of 98%.

URINALYSIS
Urine dipstick testing

- Testing the urine with dipsticks relies upon a chemical reaction occurring between the reagent in the strip and a constituent within the urine.

- Dipstick testing is useful for screening patients with possible renal tract (kidney, ureter, bladder and urethra) disease.

Following urine dipstick testing, it may be necessary to send a clean (mid-stream urine) sample to the laboratory for further diagnosis, especially when identifying an infection.

Leucocytes

- Leucocytes are white cells that may indicate urinary infection.

- A trace of leucocytes with negative nitrates, negative or trace protein and negative blood probably indicates contamination and the specimen should be repeated. The presence of glucose, albumin and some antibiotics can give a false-negative result.

Nitrites

- Most white cells in the urine produce a chemical reaction that converts nitrates into nitrites, causing the colour change on the dipstick test.

- Positive nitrate test and positive white cells are strongly suggestive of urine infection.

Urobilinogen

- This is only of importance in liver disease (*see* serum bilirubin, p. 105).

Protein

- Protein in the urine (other than a trace of protein) strongly suggests renal disease.

- A clean (mid-stream urine) sample should be sent to the laboratory to detect infection and confirm the presence of protein.

- A positive dipstick (one plus or greater) should also be sent for albumin/creatinine ratio (ACR) or protein/creatinine ratio (PCR) (depending on the test used in the local laboratory).

- SIGNIFICANT proteinuria, requiring referral, is defined as:

  - ACR of >70 OR >30 mg/mmol if haematuria is also present, *or*

  - PCR of >100 or >50 mg/mmol if haematuria is also present.

- A normal sample of urine in a small container is all that is required to quantify the ACR or PCR. A 24-hour collection of urine is not necessary.

Management of abnormal ACR/PCR

- ACR mg/mmol normal: <2.5 male, <3.5 female.
- ACR 2.5–30, optimise management of diabetes and blood pressure (BP).
- >30, refer if chronic kidney disease (CKD) 3, 4 or 5.
- >70, refer regardless of CKD.
- PCR mg/mmol normal, 4–15.
- 15–50, optimise management of diabetes and BP.
- >50, refer if CKD 3, 4 or 5.
- >100, refer regardless of CKD.

pH

- Dipstick testing gives only an approximate estimate of the acidity or alkalinity in the urine.
- Normal pH varies between 4.5 and 8.0.
- Urine pH may be important in patients with kidney stones. Altering the pH may reduce stone formation.

Blood

- A very small quantity of blood (red cells) is excreted in the urine but does not normally give a positive dipstick test.
- Blood in the urine should always be investigated further with at least a clean (mid-stream urine) specimen being sent to the laboratory to exclude infection and confirm the presence or absence of red cells.
- In women, the commonest cause of blood in the urine is menstrual blood loss.
- Other causes of blood in the urine are:
  - kidney stones
  - trauma
  - kidney infection (glomerulonephritis)
  - cancer.

Specific gravity

- Indicates the patient's urine concentration and therefore the patient's state of hydration. Specific gravity testing is not accurate or reliable.

- Normal values lie between 1,003 and 1,030.

- Specific gravity decreases with age as the kidney loses its concentrating ability.

Ketones

- These are present in dehydration and in diabetic ketoacidosis (positive ketones and positive glucose in the urine).

- Ketoacidosis (ketones and glucose both present in the urine) is a serious life-threatening condition requiring urgent blood sugar measurement and appropriate treatment (insulin).

Bilirubin

- This is not normally detectable in the urine except when liver or gallbladder disease is present.

- When the patient is jaundiced (yellow skin due to raised blood bilirubin levels), the presence of bilirubin in the urine suggests liver disease rather than other non-liver causes of jaundice.

Glucose

- Should not normally be present in the urine and occurs either because the blood sugar level is high (diabetes mellitus) or because glucose leaks from the kidney (renal glycosuria), which can occur in healthy kidneys, e.g. during pregnancy, or in diseased kidneys.

- When glucose is detected in the urine (glycosuria), a fasting blood sugar should always be performed. Diabetes is diagnosed by a fasting blood sugar >7.0 mmol/l or an HbA_{1c} >6.5 (*see* p. 140)

MICROSCOPIC HAEMATURIA

- 'Microscopic haematuria' or 'dipstick positive haematuria' may be symptomatic (with symptoms such as voiding lower urinary tract symptoms: hesitancy, frequency, urgency, dysuria) or asymptomatic (often picked up at routine medical screening).

- Urine dipstick of a fresh voided urine sample, containing no preservative, is considered a sensitive means of detecting the presence of haematuria.

- Community-based urine samples sent for microscopy have a significant false-negative rate.

- Routine microscopy for confirmation of dipstick haematuria is not necessary.

- While the sensitivity of urine dipsticks may vary from one manufacturer to another, significant microscopic haematuria is considered to be 1+ or greater. Trace haematuria can be considered negative (although it is worthwhile repeating on another occasion).

- There is no distinction in significance between non-haemolysed and haemolysed dipstick-positive haematuria.

- Significant haematuria requiring referral includes all cases of visible haematuria, all cases of symptomatic non-visible microscopic haematuria (in absence of urinary tract infection (UTI) or other transient causes such as preputial or meatal local lesions, exercise-induced haematuria, menstruation or rare causes such as myoglobulinuria) and persistent asymptomatic microscopic haematuria (two out of three dipsticks positive).

  NB: The presence of visible or microscopic haematuria should not be attributed to anticoagulant or antiplatelet therapy and patients should be investigated appropriately.

In patients with microscopic haematuria:

- Exclude UTI and/or other transient cause.

- Plasma creatinine/eGFR.

- Measure proteinuria on a random sample. Send urine for PCR or ACR on a random sample (according to local practice).

  NB: 24-hour urine collections for protein are rarely required. An approximation to the 24-hour urine protein or albumin excretion (in milligrams) is obtained by multiplying the ratio (in mg/mmol) ×10.

- Blood pressure.

Refer the following patients for a urological opinion:
- all patients with visible haematuria (any age), symptomatic microscopic haematuria (any age) or microscopic haematuria over age 40 years.

FAECAL OCCULT BLOOD (FOB)

- A FOB test may be indicative of any ulcerative or neoplastic disease of the gastrointestinal tract, including:
  - oesophageal varices
  - peptic ulcer
  - blood loss from the upper or lower gastrointestinal tract due to drugs (e.g. aspirin or non-steroidal anti-inflammatory drugs)
  - inflammatory bowel disease
  - haemorrhoids
  - benign or malignant lesions of the bowel.
- Colorectal cancer is the third-most common cancer in the UK (lung cancer, first; prostatic cancer, second), accounting for 23,000 new cases per year.
- Its frequency increases with age, the incidence doubling with each decade over 40 years.
- Two out of three people will die, while only 50% of newly diagnosed cases will have a lesion which can be totally cured by surgery.
- If colorectal cancer is diagnosed early, while restricted to the mucosa (Dukes' A), there is a 95% 5-year cure rate.
- Adenomatous polyps arising in the bowel mucosa have an increased likelihood of becoming malignant with increasing size.
- Faecal specimens should be at least 12 hours old before testing for occult blood, to allow sufficient time for haemoglobin to be converted to haematin.
- Weakly positive tests become negative within 2–4 days of storage at room temperature.
- Strongly positive stool samples still react after 10 days.
- Three stool samples, usually on consecutive days, will miss about

10% of tumours. The occult blood reaction is not specific for human haemoglobin, hence a 3-day meat-free diet is recommended prior to the test.

- Oral iron preparations can cause false-positive reactions and aspirin can cause gastrointestinal bleeding which is unrelated to gut pathology. Ascorbic acid, which is an antioxidant, interferes with the development of the colour reaction in the test.

- The following should be excluded from the diet for 3 days before collecting the stool sample for FOB testing:

  - red meat

  - cauliflower

  - broccoli

  - turnips

  - bananas

  - radish.

- Most larger polyps bleed, hence the faecal occult blood test may be useful as a screening tool. The test is safe, inexpensive and non-invasive. It does, however, have limitations – it will only detect larger polyps or cancers. As colorectal cancers only bleed intermittently, it is a relatively insensitive test and many false-negative results occur. Moreover, as other non-malignant lesions cause a positive result, it is also non-specific.

- Screening of asymptomatic people >45 years reveals 2% being positive. Of these, there is a 1:10 chance of having a carcinoma, and a 1:3 chance of having an adenoma. Of the detected tumours, >50% are early lesions, compared with only 10% of the unscreened population.

INVESTIGATION OF LEG ULCERS

- Measuring the ankle/arm pressure index with a Doppler probe (often carried out by the district nurse) enables venous ulcers (70% of leg ulcers) to be distinguished from ulcers where impaired arterial perfusion is the likely cause.

- Patients with an ankle/arm pressure index score of <0.8 should be referred for arterial assessment.

INTERPRETING DEXA SCANS IN SCREENING FOR OSTEOPOROSIS

- DEXA scanning, most accurate at the hip, is an accurate screening tool for those at risk of osteoporosis:

  - women who have had an early, natural or surgical menopause under the age of 45 years

  - women or men with a previous fragility fracture, height loss or kyphosis

  - any patient on more than 7.5 mg of steroids for more than 3 months

  - patients with secondary causes of osteoporosis, such as hyperparathyroidism, hyper- or hypothyroidism and alcohol abuse.

Interpreting DEXA scan results

- The T-score is the comparison with the young adult mean and indicates an absolute fracture risk:

  - a T-score greater than −1.0 is normal

  - a T-score between −1.0 and −2.5 indicates osteopenia and advice should be given on diet, weight-bearing exercise, smoking (stopping) and calcium and vitamin D supplements, and hormone replacement therapy may be considered

  - a T-score less than −2.5 indicates established osteoporosis and may require additional treatment.

- The Z-score is the patient's relative risk for their age:

  - a Z-score >1 indicates an increased risk of fracture.

Investigations in patients with osteoporosis before commencing treatment

- Full blood count – look at mean corpuscular volume for possible alcohol excess.

- Erythrocyte sedimentation rate to exclude myeloma.

- Liver function tests for possible alcohol excess.

- Protein electrophoresis if erythrocyte sedimentation rate is raised.

- Calcium, raised >2.65 mmol/l in hypercalcaemia, possibly due to hyperparathyroidism (raised parathyroid hormone (n = 12 – 72)) or secondary cancer (consider breast and lung).

- Testosterone, sex-hormone-binding globulin, luteinising hormone, follicle-stimulating hormone, low testosterone or free testosterone index with raised gonadotrophins, indicating hypergonadotrophic hypogonadism; low gonadotrophins indicates hypogonadotrophic hypogonadism.

- Endomysial antibodies for coeliac disease (although a 20% false-negative rate).

Chapter 7

Laboratory tests in certain clinical situations

LIVER SCREEN

(When abnormal liver function tests (LFTs) occur without reason.)

- LFT, gamma-glutamyl transferase

- Clotting studies

- Hepatitis serology

- Antinuclear antibodies (ANAs) including antimitochondrial antibodies (positive in primary biliary cirrhosis)

- Ferritin (raised in haemochromatosis)

- Ceruloplasmin (reduced in Wilson's disease)

- Immunoglobulins (may be raised in acute hepatitis and autoimmune disease)

- Abdominal ultrasound (gallstones, liver metastases)

SUSPECTED IRRITABLE BOWEL SYNDROME

- Full blood count (FBC)

- Erythrocyte sedimentation rate (ESR)/C-reactive protein (CRP)

- Tissue transglutaminase antibodies

- Stool culture sensitivity and microscopy

POLYMYALGIA RHEUMATIC (PMR)

- ESR (raised)

- CRP

- ANAs (autoimmune)

- FBC (exclude leukaemia)

- Thyroid function test (TFT) (hypo- or hyperthyroidism)

- Calcium and phosphate (hyperparathyroidism)

COELIAC ANNUAL SCREEN

(After confirmed diagnosis.)
- FBC

- Ferritin

- B$_{12}$ and folate

- Calcium and phosphate

RECURRENT MISCARRIAGE

- Clotting screen (to identify thrombophilia)

- ANAs, systemic lupus erythematosus screen (autoimmune disease)

- Anticardiolipin antibodies (antiphospholipid syndrome)

CHILDREN WITH GROWING PAINS

- FBC
- ESR/CRP
- Calcium and phosphate
- Vitamin D
- TFT
- Creatine kinase

CLAUDICATION

- FBC
- ESR/CRP
- Urea and electrolytes/LFT
- TFT
- Fasting glucose and fasting lipids

DEMENTIA SCREEN

- FBC
- ESR/CRP
- TFT
- Urea and electrolytes/LFT
- Calcium and phosphate
- Fasting glucose
- B_{12} and folate
- Clotting screen
- Syphilis serology
- Ceruloplasmin (Wilson's disease)
- HIV

PHAEOCHROMOCYTOMA

- Urinary metanephrines (noradrenaline, adrenaline, dopamine, normetadrenaline, etadrenaline), 4-hydroxy-3-methoxymandelic acid (vanillylmandelic acid), homovanillic acid, 5-hydroxyindoleacetic acid

PAGET'S DISEASE

- Bone-specific alkaline phosphatase

HIRSUTISM

- Pregnancy test
- FBC
- TFT
- Prolactin
- Free androgen index
- 24-hour urine cortisol (Cushing's disease)
- Testosterone
- 17-Alpha-hydroxyprogesterone

CHRONIC FATIGUE SYNDROME

- Urinalysis for glucose blood and protein
- FBC
- Ferritin
- B_{12} and folate
- Urea and electrolytes/LFT
- TFT
- ESR/CRP
- Autoantibodies
- Serum magnesium

- Paul–Bunnell
- Serum ACE
- Fasting glucose
- Calcium and phosphate
- Coeliac serology
- Lyme disease serology
- Hepatitis serology

UNEXPLAINED WEIGHT LOSS

- Urinalysis
- Chest X-ray
- FBC
- Ferritin/B_{12}/folate
- ESR/CRP
- Lactic dehydrogenase (>500 is associated with likely malignant cause)
- Urea and electrolytes/LFT
- TFT
- Fasting glucose
- Coeliac serology
- Faecal occult blood (if available)

MYELOMA

- FBC (often a normochromic normocytic anaemia)
- ESR (usually >30, sometimes much higher)
- CRP (often raised)
- Urea and electrolytes/LFT
- Uric acid (often raised)

- Total protein albumin and serum globulins (often <19 or >48 g/l)

- Serum protein electrophoresis

- Calcium (adjusted calcium often >2.65 mmol/l with low parathyroid hormone and no known primary cancer

ERECTILE DYSFUNCTION
- FBC

- Ferritin (haemochromatosis)

- Urea and electrolytes/LFT

- Fasting glucose and cholesterol

- Prolactin

- Luteinising hormone (to distinguish between primary and secondary hypogonadism)

- TFT

- Early-morning serum testosterone/sex-hormone-binding globulin

TINNITUS
- FBC

- Urea and electrolytes/LFT (metabolic disorders can cause tinnitus)

MALARIA
- FBC, thick and thin film (looking for parasites) (blood film can be taken at any time, not just when the patient is febrile)

- Malaria rapid antigen test (usually available within 1 hour)

- Blood culture for typhoid and other

- Bacteraemia

- Urea and electrolytes/LFT

- Random blood glucose

SYSTEMIC LUPUS ERYTHEMATOSUS

- FBC – normochromic normocytic anaemia is common, as is thrombocytopenia (<100) and leucopenia (<4 × 10^9/l)

- ESR (often high)

- CRP (often normal)

- ANA

- Anti-double-stranded DNA antibodies (lupus anticoagulant, anticardiolipin antibodies)

OSTEOPOROSIS

- FBC

- Urea and electrolytes/LFT

- ESR

- Calcium and phosphate

- Testosterone in men

- Follicle-stimulating hormone in women (under age 55 years)

PRURITUS

- Urinalysis (for glucose blood and protein)

- FBC (anaemia, polycythaemia, leucopenia, thrombocytopenia)

- ESR (may be raised in myeloma lymphoma or other malignancy)

- Ferritin (low ferritin causes pruritus)

- Urea and electrolytes/LFT (renal failure can cause itching, as does obstructive biliary disease and chronic liver disease)

- TFT (pruritus may occur in hypo- or hyperthyroidism)

- Fasting glucose (pruritus can occur in diabetes)

- Calcium (raised calcium in myeloma can cause pruritus)

HYPERTENSION

- Urinalysis (for blood protein or glucose)
- FBC (raised mean corpuscular volume may suggest excess alcohol, polycythaemia may suggest heavy cigarette smoking)
- urea and electrolytes (high sodium may suggest primary aldosteronism, low potassium may suggest primary or secondary aldosteronism; hypokalaemia, hypernatraemia in Conn's syndrome)
- Estimated glomerular filtration rate
- Urinary metanephrines
- Urinary cortisol or 0900 hours serum cortisol measurement

GYNAECOMASTIA

- FBC
- LFT
- TFT
- Prolactin
- Testosterone and serum sex-hormone-binding globulin

UNEXPLAINED LOSS OF CONSCIOUSNESS

- FBC
- Urea and electrolytes/LFT
- Fasting or random glucose
- Calcium and phosphate

MONOCLONAL GAMMOPATHY OF UNDETERMINED SIGNIFICANCE

- FBC
- Urea and electrolytes/LFT
- Paraproteins

PATIENT TAKING A STATIN

- Urea and electrolytes/LFT (or alanine transferase)
- Lipid profile (fasting or non-fasting)

HYPERPARATHYROIDISM

- Urea and electrolytes/LFT
- Calcium and phosphate
- Vitamin D

CHRONIC KIDNEY DISEASE (CKD) MONITORING

Frequency depends upon severity of CKD – for example, in CKD 3, monitor the following 6-monthly.

- FBC
- Urea and electrolytes/LFT
- Calcium and phosphate
- Urine protein/creatinine ratio

INVESTIGATIONS FOLLOWING AN UNEXPLAINED LOW-RISK DEEP VEIN THROMBOSIS

- FBC
- Urea and electrolytes
- Calcium
- Chest X-ray

(All to exclude occult malignancy.)

Index

CPD with Radcliffe

You can now use a selection of our books to achieve CPD (Continuing Professional Development) points through directed reading.

We provide a free online form and downloadable certificate for your appraisal portfolio. Look for the CPD logo and register with us at: www.radcliffehealth.com/cpd

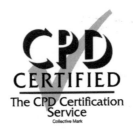